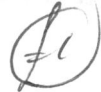

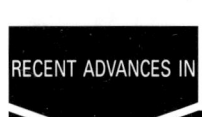
RECENT ADVANCES IN

Anaesthesia and Analgesia

Edited by

A. P. Adams MB BS PhD FRCA FANZCA FFARACS DA
Professor of Anaesthetics, University of London;
Honorary Consultant Anaesthetist, Guy's and St Thomas' Hospitals,
and Bethlem Royal and Maudsley Hospital Neurosurgical Unit, London, UK

J. N. Cashman BSc MB BS BA PhD FRCA
Department of Anaesthetics, St George's Hospital, London, UK

NUMBER NINETEEN

CHURCHILL LIVINGSTONE
EDINBURGH LONDON MADRID MELBOURNE MILAN NEW YORK AND TOKYO 1995

CHURCHILL LIVINGSTONE
Medical Division of Pearson Professional UK Limited

Distributed in the United States of America by
Churchill Livingstone Inc., 650 Avenue of the Americas,
New York, N.Y. 10011, and by associated companies,
branches and representatives throughout the world.

First published 1995

ISBN 0443 053065
ISSN 0309-2305

British Library Cataloguing in Publication Data
A catalogue record for this book is available from the British
Library

Library of Congress Cataloging in Publication Data
is available

The
publisher's
policy is to use
**paper manufactured
from sustainable forests**

Produced by Longman Singapore Publisher Pte Ltd
Printed in Singapore

Contents

Foreword

Dr R S Atkinson and *Recent Advances in Anaesthesia and Analgesia* – an appreciation

The last volume – the 18th – was the final one for my senior co-editor Dr Dick Atkinson who was about to retire from clinical practice. I interviewed him at the end of 1994 regarding the series. He recalls that the sixth edition of *Recent Advances in Anaesthesia and Analgesia*, published in 1945, was the first serious anaesthetic book he bought when he began his career in anaesthesia at the beginning of 1952. The first seven editions, which appeared at regular intervals since the first in 1932, had all been written by Dr Christopher Langton Hewer of St. Bartholmew's Hospital. He was one of the leading anaesthetists of his day, though known universally (unofficially) as 'Gloomy' owing to his propensity for relating untoward happenings in other hospitals. I first got to know him when I wrote to him for permission to reproduce some material which had appeared in *Recent Advances* and nothing was too much trouble to help a young doctor.

Dick Atkinson became interested in writing when still at school in the war years. In the VIth form he studied physics, chemistry and mathematics, but after one year decided he wanted to become a doctor although there was no one medical in his family. This meant that he had to give up mathematics and take up biology for the Higher School Certificate Examination. The first response from his Headmaster was that 'it was out of the question', but perseverance eventually won. The next problem lay in the fact that the best schoolteachers had left for military duties and with only one year to go to the examination Atkinson decided he would have to do a lot of work on his own. This he did by making a précis (or synopsis) of important chapters in the books. Then a superb biology teacher suddenly arrived in the school who was an enormous help. The Higher School Certificate successfully passed, he stayed on at school for two extra terms to sit for a scholarship examination to Cambridge University after which he was awarded an Exhibition to Trinity Hall, gaining more than 80% in biology though only 30% in chemistry.

Atkinson moved to St. Bartholomew's Hospital, London, in 1948 to pursue his clinical studies, which included one month in anaesthesia, where he first met Langton Hewer. Qualifying in medicine in 1951, Atkinson was unsuccessful in his application for a House Physician post at the North Middlesex Hospital. He never held a House Surgeon post, there being no requirement by the General Medical Council for a one year pre-registration period in those days. He then applied for a second post at Bart's and was appointed a House Officer in the Department of Anaesthetics, working with the units operating at Hill End Hospital, St. Albans, where they had moved during the war years but still not returned to the mother site. Atkinson then had second thoughts about this and consulted the then Dean of the Medical School, Dr Charles Harris, who could only advise him not to accept a post he was unhappy about. Nevertheless, others suggested a short time in anaesthesia could do no harm and after some thought Atkinson accepted the post, which was only for a duration of six months!

The next problem was that his North Middlesex post did not end until six weeks after the one at Hill End was due to start. However, he was lucky to be allowed to take the last two weeks of his medical post as annual leave and to start the anaesthesia one a month late. When he arrived at Hill End on the first day of the month, he was greeted by Dr Hewer with the remark, 'I'm sorry this is not the job you wanted'.

Nevertheless, Atkinson found he enjoyed anaesthesia. He found a facility for the work and had stimulating teachers. The spectrum of work was interesting since orthopaedics, ENT, cardiothoracic and neurosurgery were housed at Hill End which also accommodated the plastic surgery unit that later moved to Northwood. The main part of Hill End Hospital looked after the psychiatric patients who were no concern of St. Bartholomew's.

In the early 1950s there were relatively few textbooks in anaesthesia, Those Atkinson read were Hewer's *Recent Advances in Anaesthesia and Analgesia*, Lee's *Synopsis of Anaesthesia* and Frankis Evans' *Modern Practice in Anaesthesia* supplemented by his preclinical books for the Primary DA examination which he sat for and passed at the end of what had become a full year in anaesthesia at Hill End. From then on a career in anaesthesia became a certainty. Atkinson was a Senior House Officer at the Prince of Wales Hospital in Tottenham and then spent two years National Service in the Royal Army Medical Corps during which time he passed the first examination for the Final FFARCS (Fellow in the Faculty of Anaesthetists of the Royal College of Surgeons of England) held in December 1953. On demobilisation he held Registrar and Senior Registrar posts at St. Bartholomew's Hospital (much of the time spent at Hill End) which included one year at the Hospital of the University of Pennsylvania in Philadelphia and one year at Chase Farm Hospital, Enfield.

In 1961 Atkinson took up a Consultant Anaesthetist post at Southend Hospital, Essex where he became a colleague of Dr Alfred Lee. Dr Langton Hewer was meantime still working on *Recent Advances in Anaesthesia and Analgesia*. After the seventh edition in 1953 he shared the labours with Dr Alfred Lee for the 8th edition in 1957. Up to this point all the writing had been undertaken by the authors themselves. From the ninth edition onwards the editor(s) invited contributions from distinguished specialists. Atkinson contributed a chapter on 'Monitoring' for the tenth edition (1967) and one on the 'Place of the anaesthetist in the Intensive Care Unit' for the 11th edition in 1972. The first ten editions were published by Messrs. J. and A. Churchill Ltd, a forerunner of the present publishers Churchill Livingstone. Langton Hewer invited Atkinson as his co-editor for the twelfth edition of 1967 and subsequent editions. This edition was noteworthy for doubling up as the Spring edition (vol. 16, No. 1) of *International Anesthesiology Clinics of North America*. The thirteenth edition (1979) was the first edition published as a softback version in which A. P. Adams and J. D. Henville from Oxford were invited to contribute a joint chapter on flexible pipelines and anaesthetic breathing systems. By 1982 the series was fifty years old with the publication of the fourteenth edition and this was marked by the editorship changing to Atkinson and Hewer, rather than Hewer and Atkinson, to reflect the balance of the labour involved. Langton Hewer wrote a chapter '50 Years on' to commemorate this issue. When Langton Hewer finally bowed out, Atkinson invited me to join him as his co-editor and the fifteenth edition appeared in 1985. The sixteenth, seventeenth and eighteenth editions appeared in 1989, 1992, and 1994 respectively.

Dick Atkinson has thus been an editor of *Recent Advances in Anaesthesia and Analgesia* for seven editions extending over almost 20 years. He is a well-known author and editor of many other works in anaesthesia of course, but it should be placed on record the immense effort and dedication to this series.

Anthony P. Adams
London, 1995

Preface

Recent Advances in Anaesthesia and Analgesia is now in its sixty-third year of publication. Dr Richard Atkinson has retired as senior editor and Dr Jeremy Cashman has now joined the team. This edition continues to present reviews of important topics for busy practising anaesthetists. Contributions have come from distinguished colleagues in Europe as well as from various parts of the UK.

The press is always ready to report hospital mistakes, for example, problem areas of wakefulness during general anaesthesia and of pain control. Dr Green is a psychologist who is internationally known to anaesthetists through his writings and lectures. He brings us up-to-date on the subject of human error that is of vital importance in our specialty and currently a major topic of interest. Doctors taken to court tend not to fare well without good hospital notes and Dr de Mello and Professor Adams consider anaesthetic records which are a most active area of interest by various bodies including SCATA – the Society for Computing and Technology in Anaesthesia – and a current working party of the Royal College of Anaesthetists. The subject of minimally invasive surgery has also been in the news and the Royal College of Surgeons of England now organises training for surgeons on simulators. The anaesthetic aspects are equally important and are considered by Dr Brichant. 'Mother in agony during baby op' has also hit the headlines recently and the subject of providing good pain relief with epidural or spinal block, or general anaesthesia if necessary, for maternity cases is brought right up-to-date by Dr Lyons. Every anaesthetist should be proficient in fibreoptic intubation: Dr Pearce and his colleagues at Guy's Hospital have organised a national course on this subject for 7 years and he presents a state of the art view. The solution to the problem of reliably detecting awareness during general anaesthesia continues to exert the minds of the experts, and Dr Pomfrett presents the concept of RR intervals that has the attraction of being based upon conventionally recorded physiological variables. Postoperative nausea and vomiting continue to distress many of our patients and Drs Matson and Palazzo review this subject in the context of new drugs available. Pain control in children – or rather the lack of it – has also been 'newsworthy' and Drs Murdoch and Cashman bring this subject to our attention. Non-acute pain has not been considered in depth in the series for some years and so Dr Justins has reviewed this topic. Septic shock, and its treatment, has also been in the news and we are grateful to Professor Vincent for giving us the benefit of his extensive knowledge. Finally, the Royal College of Anaesthetists has this year decided to move away from a three-part to a two-part examination: this first part will be called the *Primary* and the second part the *Final*. We are grateful to Dr Hewitt for her presentation regarding the mode of new examinations.

The editors hope the reader will find these chapters informative and helpful whether he or she is in the trainee grade, an examination candidate or an established practitioner. We are mindful that some do not have ready access to books and journals especially in remote parts. We are most grateful to the contributors for their effort and to the publishers for their help and support.

London   A.P.A.
1995   J.N.C.

Contributors

Professor A P Adams MB BS PhD FRCA FANZCA FFA RACS DA
Professor of Anaesthetics, United Medical and Dental Schools, Guy's and St Thomas's Hospitals, London, UK. Honorary Consultant Anaesthetist, Guy's and St Thomas' Hospitals NHS Trust, Royal Bethlem and Maudsley NHS Trust, London, UK

Dr J-F Brichant
Spécialiste des Hôpitaux, Départment d'Anesthesie et Réanimation, CHU de Liège, Hôpital de la Citadelle, Liège, Belgium

Dr J N Cashman BSc MB BS BA FRCA
Consultant Anaesthetist, St George's Hospital, London, UK

Lt Col W F de Mello RAMC
BSc MBBS FRCA DRCOG Dip IMCRCS (Ed)
Director of Intensive Care, Cambridge Military Hospital, Aldershot, UK. Senior Lecturer in Anaesthetics and Resuscitation (Army), Royal Army Medical College, London, UK

Dr R Green BSc CPsychol FRAeS AFBPsS
Chief Scientist, DRA Centre for Human Sciences, Farnborough, Hants, UK. Honorary Professor, University of Wales. Visiting Professor, Cranfield University

Dr P B Hewitt MB BS FRCA DA
Consultant Anaesthetist, Department of Anaesthetics, Guy's Hospital and the Maudsley Neurosurgical Unit, Honorary Senior Lecturer, United Medical and Dental Schools, London, UK

Dr D Justins MB BS FRCA
Consultant in Anaesthesia and Pain Management, St Thomas' Hospital, London, UK

Dr G Lyons FRCA
Consultant Obstetric Anaesthetist, St James's University Hospital, Leeds, UK

Dr A Matson MB BS FRCA
Consultant Anaesthetist, West Middlesex Hospital, Surrey, UK

Dr L Murdoch MB BS FRCA
Consultant Paediatric Anaethetist, St George's Hospital, London, UK

Dr M Palazzo MB ChB FRCP FRCA MD
Senior Lecturer and Honorary Consultant in Anaesthesia, Department of Anaesthetics, Charing Cross Hospital, London, UK

Dr A C Pearce FFA RCS Eng
Consultant Anaesthetist, Department of Anaesthetics, Guy's Hospital, London, UK

Dr C J D Pomfrett BSc PhD
Lecturer in Neurophysiology Applied to Anaesthesia, University Department of Anaesthesia, Manchester University, Manchester, UK

Professor J-L Vincent MD PhD
Department of Intensive Care, University Hospital Brussels, Belgium

The psychology of human error

R. Green

It is well recognized that many, probably the majority of, accidents in anaesthesia arise from human error. [1-6] In some studies 75% of intraoperative cardiac arrests appeared to be caused by preventable anaesthetic errors. [7] Another study estimated that inadequate patient observation alone contributed to one-third of deaths. [8] There is a notable similarity between these statistics and those in aviation, where about three-quarters of all air carrier accidents are similarly attributable to operator error. This is not the only similarity between anaesthesia and flying: both require the interaction of human beings with sophisticated technological equipment and the operation of this equipment in well defined ways. Both also require, however, that the human operator, pilot or anaesthetist, should be able to make an overall subjective assessment of a multivariate situation in which some of the variables may be relatively poorly, and only qualitatively, defined. For example, the anaesthetist must assess the physical appearance of the patient and the pilot must make subjective assessments of the state of the weather. In addition, both anaesthetist and pilot are required to possess certain motor skills that may be acquired only through practice, to interact with other individuals in teams, and to form a component in a large organization.

There is potential in all of the areas outlined above for error to occur. The reason for drawing these parallels between anaesthesia and flying is because there has probably been more research into pilot error than into error in any other profession, and there may be procedures in place in flying that could usefully be adapted to anaesthesia. [9,10] It is also probably true that aircraft presently offer more advanced interfaces to the operator than anaesthetic machines, and thus may signal problems yet to arrive in anaesthesia.

MENTAL MODELS

It is a prerequisite of most behaviour that the anaesthetist has a mental model of his situation and environment. [11] It goes without saying that our situational mental model (our internal representation of the real world situation in which we find ourselves) is based on sensory input. Thus the page

that is presently in front of you is projected on the retina as a white trape-
zium containing black marks, but by the time that the sensory data have
been delivered to the brain and compared with our stored experiences, you
will have not only an internal model of the external object (a book), but this
will have been placed within the context of your overall knowledge (the
book is about anaesthesia and you are an anaesthetist sitting at home read-
ing it). Pilots call the possession of an accurate high level model 'situational
awareness'.[12]

It is obviously important for an anaesthetist to have good overall situational
awareness, but there are 3 main ways in which it can break down. If we have
strong expectations about a situation then these expectations may lead us
to generate a model of which we are confident, but that is wrong. To give
a trivial example, if a class of physiology students is shown this group of
letters 'P_Y__OLOGY' they will report seeing the word 'physiology' with
some letters missing, whereas a psychology class will report the same but
for the word 'psychology'. This example is not as far removed from real life
as it may appear, since we are constantly presented with sensory data that
are far from perfect or complete, yet we make good situational models from
them. Occasionally, we make the error of allowing this model to be based
more on our expectations than on sensory data (i.e. 'jumping to a conclusion') but there is an even more important possible subsequent effect that
I will refer to as 'confirmation bias'.[13] This refers to the fact that once we
have generated a mental model of a situation, we usually tend to behave in
ways that seek to confirm that model rather than in ways that attempt to
test it, the only way of doing this being to try to gain 'disconfirming' information from the world. The safety hazard of this natural behaviour is
obvious and, interestingly, the phrase 'The exception proves the rule' does
not mean that finding an exception to a general rule is some form of
perverse demonstration of the rule, since 'prove' here is used in the sense
of 'test' (as in 'proving ground') to mean that the exception (the disconfirming evidence) tests the rule.

Unfortunately, as observed above, we do not generally tend to behave in
ways that test our situational model, but the opposite. In a well known
aviation incident, a Boeing 747 was approaching Nairobi when the air traffic controller cleared the aircraft to 'seven, five, zero, zero' feet. The crew
failed to hear the 'seven' because of poor communications quality, so sensed
only the last three digits. Nevertheless, because they were expecting a clearance to a few thousand feet, both pilots believed that they had been cleared
to five, zero, zero, **zero** feet. This initial error of expectation was then com-
pounded by confirmation bias as a number of automatic warnings that should
have alerted the pilots to their real situation were treated as faulty warnings
by the crew. Even when the aircraft broke cloud very close to the ground,
the captain treated the sight of the unexpectedly close ground as a visual
illusion. Analogous errors are plainly possible, and have certainly occurred
in anaesthesia. Clinical observations such as visualizing cyanosis can be

ambiguous and open to the generation of an inappropriate model and this may be exacerbated by equipment displays that are not sufficiently easy to read.

Failure to test the basic situational model may also be observed in those who may inadvertently have given an incorrect injection because of an ampoule swap or inadvertently performed an oesophageal intubation. Such individuals may well not test or question their basic model when the patient begins to show signs of distress, and instead look for failures in the anaesthetic machine or connections.

Although there can be no doubt that the jump to an inappropriate conclusion followed by confirmation bias is a powerful and important cause of human error, little has ever been achieved by way of prevention. I believe that it is possible to develop ways of training that provide ways of enabling operators to recognize such experience and these are returned to below.

The second way in which situational models may cause problems is when the sensory data are accurately perceived, but do not enable the formation of a mental model because they are insufficient or, more likely, because the operator has not experienced the situation before and therefore possesses neither any expectations of it nor any cognitive framework within which to accommodate it. In such situations the operator will be in good contact with his environment but not understand what is happening. They may be resolved only through thinking and reasoning, and this subject is also dealt with below.

The last type of mental model failure occurs when there is an inappropriate distribution of attention that simply prevents the construction of an adequate model. The classic example of this type of situation in aviation is where the pilot identifies a problem with the aircraft, gives his whole attention to solving it, but flies into the ground because of a failure of overall situational awareness.[14] This was precisely the case in the accident in which a Lockheed TriStar crashed into the Florida Everglades while all of the crew members were trying to change a cockpit light bulb, and also regularly occurs in anaesthesia. Indeed, there is probably much greater scope for its occurrence in anaesthesia since a single anaesthetist will be required both to deal with any problem that arises and maintain good awareness of the principal task of maintaining the patient in good condition. Good basic training, and regular recurrent training, in dealing with problems and emergencies are plainly **essential** if such occurrences are to be minimized.[15]

AUTOMATIC BEHAVIOURS

The behaviour of individual operators is sometimes divided into three categories that are loosely based on Rasmussen's model,[16,17] and for present purposes, may be described as **automatic behaviours, drills and procedures**, and **reasoned behaviours**. It is a great but reasonable simplification to regard these behaviours as capable of division into those that are consciously controlled (the drills and reasoned behaviours) and those that proceed autonomously or automatically, usually after conscious initiation. For example, we may decide to walk, hit a golf ball, or throw a switch, but once the decision is made the action is carried out without conscious intervention. Indeed it is a characteristic of such 'skills' that once they are well acquired, conscious intervention can spoil their execution. Quite complex behaviours may be carried out in this automatic way as long as they are well practised, and it is commonplace for skilled drivers to realise that they have arrived at their destination without any recollection of the journey because their consciousness was devoted to considering some non-driving matter while they followed a habitual route. It is fortunate that we are able to behave in this way, since the 'channel capacity' for conscious decision making is so limited that it would be very constraining if we were not able to carry out several automatic behaviours at the same time as one under conscious control. Generally, good priority management exists to ensure that the appropriate behaviour receives conscious control (for example, we may talk and drive simultaneously, but when an emergency is presented on the road, the conversation ceases immediately as full conscious decision making is given to the driving task).

A number of types of error may occur here, however.[18-20] First, the correct decision may be made but the wrong automatic behaviour engaged (e.g. a correct decision may be made to increase the flow of gas A only for the flow of gas B to be in fact increased instead). In such instances the behaviour that is executed in error is almost always similar to the intended behaviour, but the danger is that the error usually goes consciously unnoticed, and the operator believes him or herself to have taken the correct action. The second type of such failure is sometimes referred to as 'environmental capture'. If a series of actions is always carried out in a certain set of circumstances, then these actions may be carried out habitually even when inappropriate. This can have ludicrous results if somebody who is used to going to the operating theatre, getting changed, and scrubbing up goes to the theatre only to collect some notes but finds that he or she has changed and scrubbed up anyway. Such environmental capture can be dangerous, however, if the driver of a double decker bus drives along his habitual single decker route under a low bridge (several such examples exist), or an anaesthetist (even though previously aware of a patient's particular sensitivity) uses a habitual anaesthetic technique rather than that appropriate to the special instance. The third main way in which automatic behaviours fail is through a lack of critical perceptual appraisal. It appears as though the perceptual information needed to drive automatic behaviours is dealt with relatively uncritically so that similar objects may be substituted for one another. I myself have attempted, while mentally distracted, to clean my teeth with 'Germolene', and a colleague informed me of a more distressing confusion between 'Deep Heat' and 'KY Jelly'. More dangerous, of course, is the possibility of such a substitution occurring between two similar ampoules, and this clearly occurs on a daily basis.[21]

It is sometimes suggested that in order to minimize such events, operators should train themselves to make all actions in stages with conscious intervention before final execution. Thus, in operating a switch, the sequence would be (1) make decision, (2) grasp switch, (3) check for correctness (i.e. conscious intervention), (4) operate switch. Ideally, of course, the check would not be carried out by the operator but by a third party, and such checks of one pilot's behaviour by the other on the flight deck are commonplace. It may well be that there is much greater scope for independent checking, for example of correctness of all injections, in anaesthesia and this should probably be considered. In addition, circumstances demanding behaviour other than habitual behaviour should be well flagged with the use of warnings, red wristbands and so on. On flight decks there are relatively few switches that can cause disaster through their inadvertent operation, and these are made conspicuous and well guarded. It may well be that there would be a similarly limited number of substances that are critically hazardous when injected and, if so, their containers should be made similarly conspicuous.

DRILLS AND PROCEDURES

It can be argued that the single most important reason why flying, an activity of obvious intrinsic danger, is as safe as it is, is the 'proceduralization' of the flying task. Forty years ago, a pilot required to fly to a given destination would have had a great deal of freedom over how he set about the flight and how, for example, he planned his approach to land given the nature of the airfield, the state of the wind, the availability of navigational aids, and the presence of hazards, such as high ground. The anaesthetist probably still has such freedom in deciding how to approach his task, but flying is now much more constrained. Whereas the anaesthetist may have no explicit anaesthetic plan, the pilot in a large airline will be provided with a computerised flight plan in which all of the factors that he would once have had to consider for himself will have been taken into account. Moreover, when it comes to making his approach to land, all possible ways of executing an approach to a given airfield will have already been considered and his job will be to fly the preplanned approach profile relevant to the conditions of the day. Moreover, all conceivable aircraft failures will have been anticipated in advance and drills will have been developed to deal with them. If the drill or procedure demands rapid execution (e.g. an engine failure during take off) the pilot will be required to be able to execute it from memory, otherwise the use of flight reference cards and checklists ensure the standard execution of the drill. All pilots will have been schooled in these drills and will be refreshed and assessed in their use at intervals of six months in the flight simulator. Some airlines have gone further in using a data recorder in the aircraft and daily computerized analysis of the data from this recorder to ensure that the pilots have not departed from standard procedures. Even in the absence of a simulator, however, it has been shown that 'mental rehearsal' of drills can be effective and is probably to be recommended.

The development of standard procedures and checklists, the simulator training of pilots in their use, and the checking of pilots to ensure continued competence and adherence to standards have been outstandingly successful in aviation. Although attempts have been made in each of these areas in anaesthesia,[22] none of them is anything like so well developed, so formalized, or so widespread as in aviation. There may be many reasons for this, but I would venture to suggest just two. The first is that proceduralization of a job and the regular competence testing of those carrying it out smacks of 'deprofessionalizing' it. 'Professionals' will argue that the situations that present themselves in their jobs are complex, differ from one occasion to another, and thus require careful individual evaluation. This may well be so to some extent and represents a good case for keeping intelligent, knowledgeable, and well trained people doing the job, but this does not represent an argument for failing to adopt standard procedures for all situations and emergencies that can be anticipated. Interestingly, these arguments were once made with regard to the pilot's job, yet no pilot today would regard standard operating procedures and competence testing as anything other than obviously essential. The second reason may be associated with the fact that commercial aviation has a regulatory authority that is independent of any commercial interest in aviation or any pilot interest group. This authority lays down standards for airline training and checking, approves the operating procedures of an airline and, if dissatisfied, can prevent the individual pilot or entire airline from operating. By comparison, the regulation of all medical specialties, essentially by peer organizations that may also act as practitioner interest groups, appears weaker and more informal.

THINKING AND REASONING

It is obvious, however, that not all situations may be anticipated, that there can never be a standard procedure for every event, and thus that system operators of all types will be required, on occasions, to solve problems as and when they arise. Some of the issues concerned with problem solving have already been addressed in the discussion on situational awareness above, since a prerequisite for solving a problem is an accurate overall appreciation of it. It has been pointed out, however, that when solving a problem or deciding what action to take in a novel set of circumstances inferences are probably made from the operator's basic knowledge base, and high level analogies are sought that enable the execution of a behaviour that seems most appropriate: the operator may try to convert an unrecognized situation into one for which he or she has a solution available. It may be argued that making a large part of the operator's task rule-based may thus make the operator inflexible in dealing with novel situations since he or she may lose the capacity to think of innovative solutions, and become even more reliant on behaving in preplanned and prelearned ways.

In aviation, it has been argued that simulator training and checks that are exclusively based on standard operating procedures have not addressed the issue of problem solving, and attempts are now being made to introduce what is termed Line Orientated Flying Training (LOFT) in order to rectify this situation. The object is to run a simulator exercise (though a simulator may not be essential for such problem solving training) in which obvious and clear cut emergencies are avoided, but in which situations, often multivariate in nature, develop and require high level thought and decision making for solution. Frequently a unique solution will not exist, the object being to train the operator to develop the skills necessary to assess situations as objectively and accurately as possible, to make the fullest use of the data available in generating a solution, not to ignore data that are inconvenient to the chosen solution path (i.e. to avoid confirmation bias),[23] to make the fullest use of available resources and information sources available, and to contemplate ways of reviewing and testing both the situational model and the solution generated. Frequently such exercises are video-taped for subsequent debriefing and discussion. Unfortunately, as is true for many types of training, it is difficult to demonstrate its effectiveness in terms of a safety improvement but, since problem solving is a skill, it is reasonable to assume that it will benefit from the sort of practice that is likely to provide operators with strategies (rather than drills) for dealing with novel situations.

STRESS AND FATIGUE

The foregoing has dealt with behaviours associated with the individual, but all of these behaviours are likely to be affected by the presence of stress. There are many models relating stress to human performance[24-26] but there are probably three categories of stress that are likely to affect the anaesthetist. The first category of stress, acute reactive stress, arises from the occurrence of a critical incident or emergency. It is well recognized that whereas the autonomic response associated with such stress is well adapted to producing physical activity, it is distinctly less helpful in conditions where a more cerebral response is required. An excessive concentration of attention on the apparent cause of the problem and a failure to utilize more peripheral, but possibly important, information is a characteristic in these circumstances. Simulation may well be of benefit here in two ways; first in providing the operator with a procedure to follow if the emergency is of a type that could be anticipated and, second, in habituating the affective response to the emergency and making it more likely that the operator will remain calm when the event really occurs. Many pilots who experience an engine fire when airborne report that it was not particularly worrying since it was just like the simulator.

The second category of stress comprises environmental and work-related effects.[27,28] The operating theatre may be rather noisy and thermally uncomfortable, but such factors are unlikely to reach troublesome proportions. Fatigue is an important issue, however, and may be either work-induced as a result of a long duty times or be produced by working at a time that is inappropriate to the individual's circadian rhythm (usually by working at night). Well practised skills and drills seem relatively insensitive to the effects of fatigue, but it appears that there is a general reduction in cognitive or mental resources resulting in poor judgements, problem solving, and decision making. It is notable that there is a disproportionately large number of motorway accidents between 2 am and 6 am, and the bad decisions at Chernobyl and Three Mile Island were also made at this time – the lowest ebb of the human circadian rhythm. There is an extensive literature on these effects[29–34] and flight duty time legislation recognizes and controls both of them (in addition to effects produced by crossing time zones). This legislation is constantly revised and is a major source of contention between pilot associations, airline managements, and regulatory authorities. Presently, new regulations are being enacted on a European basis and these have attracted much interest and criticism within aviation.[35,36]

Although these regulations in aviation may be difficult to generate, there is complete acceptance by all sides of the industry that they are essential for safety. They are thus not a code of conduct or advisory guidelines, but mandatory. It is difficult to see why there should not be parallel rules in those areas of medical practice, such as anaesthesia, where similar problems may occur, and it is difficult to believe that it would not be in the interest of patient safety for such rules to be introduced. This should be regarded as a system problem and is returned to below.

The third category of stress that may affect the anaesthetist is that of life or domestic stress. Both pilots and anaesthetists have life styles that revolve around a job that may present conflict with home and family life. Although there are demonstrated relationships between the degree of life stress and health and well being[25] there is little by way of demonstrated relationship between life stress and error. There is anecdotal evidence, and common sense suggest that domestic problems and stress cannot be completely divorced from professional activities, but the question, of course, is what may be done about it.

There are three basic techniques dealing with those chronic stresses that may arise from an unsatisfactory work or home environment.[26] The first is 'cognitive coping' and consists of confronting the situation mentally (possibly with the help of a friend or colleague) and coming to a realistic and as objective as possible appreciation of it. The problem may not seem so bad when it is tackled rationally. The second is termed 'action coping' and is self evident in meaning: worry about an exam may be reduced by doing some revision, or the stress of working for an impossible boss may be eliminated by changing job. Third is 'symptom directed' coping and usually refers to the use of alcohol and drugs in order to alleviate the anxiety and depression that may be associated with stress. Anaesthetists are plainly not immune from this last form of coping (indeed they may be especially susceptible), but will realise that although it may have some short term utility, its long term ill advisedness is self-evident.

WORKING IN TEAMS

Although some pilots and anaesthetists may work essentially alone, most will co-operate with others of related skills in a small team.[37] Although there are several exercises in which the team procedures developed for flight decks[36-39] have been applied to operating theatres, it should be borne in mind that these teams are different from one another in several important respects. Rank, seniority, and authority are made quite explicit on the flight deck (emblems of rank are displayed, the captain sits in the left seat, and so on) but in a theatre all are dressed identically. More importantly, the aircraft captain is always in command, whereas in an operating theatre, the individual who is giving instructions may vary depending on the nature of the problem. In aircraft the actual functions undertaken (either flying the aircraft or carrying out non-flying aspects of the flight) will be swapped from captain to first officer and vice versa but in a theatre the surgeon, anaesthetist, and nurse have defined tasks that are not (at least, not normally) interchanged.[40]

For these reasons, much of the expertise that has been developed to assist flight deck teams to make correct joint decisions may not be relevant in anaesthesia, but there are probably some basic social psychological effects that should be recognized. The first is that team members and especially leaders can be regarded in terms of the extent to which they are task and goal orientated and the extent to which they have an interpersonal or emotional orientation. Ideally, all team members will recognize that there are times, usually when things are going well, when showing consideration for other individuals and their problems is appropriate (the democratic style), and other times (especially when a difficulty or an emergency presents itself) when task demands over-ride the requirement for interpersonal consideration (the autocratic style).[26] Difficulties arise, of course, when an individual is either too demanding and inconsiderate of his colleagues when it would be reasonable to be otherwise or when, conversely, an individual fails to assert proper task leadership because he is too concerned about upsetting his colleagues. It is particularly difficult, of course, for a relatively junior member of a team to make demands related to his function within the team of a more senior or more dominant member who may even have conflicting goals. These problems are presently addressed in flying by subjecting pilots to courses in Flight Deck Management or Crew Resource Management,[39] and airlines in the United Kingdom are now compelled to run such courses by the regulatory authority.

The ways in which people interact are naturally complex and involve many social psychological effects that determine, for example, our likelihood of complying with the request of another, our likelihood of conforming to the views of a group even when they vary with our personal views, the likelihood of a group making a more extreme decision than any of its members would have made individually but, despite this, some simple and obvious guidelines to group decision making may be offered. These revolve around the fact that, generally speaking, even though only one member of a group may solve a problem correctly, the other members are likely to recognize the best solution when it is presented to them. This makes it crucial that, when group problem solving, all members of the group should be enabled to submit their views, ideas, and solutions.

Without training, a group leader may believe that the best way of exercising leadership is to outline his or her view of and solution to a problem as a basis for discussion among other group members.[26] The difficulty of this approach is that if a junior member of the group has a better solution, he or she may be reluctant to air it since to do so may appear to be contradicting or scoring a point off the leader. The best way for the leader to behave is: first, to ask the group members for their view of the nature of the problem to ensure that no aspect of it is ignored; second, to summarize these views to obtain agreement on problem definition; third, to ask for candidate solutions and gain group agreement on the best; fourth, if necessary make a choice between competing solutions or courses of action explaining, if possible, the reasons for the choice.

It is also important for all members of a group to appreciate that it is their responsibility fully to air their views when called upon to do so, but to conform to the joint decision of the group once this has been made, unless they believe that some hazard or danger has gone unrecognized. Furthermore group members should not allow personal feelings to intrude into their contribution to a group and should always bear in mind the overall goal, normally the safety of the patient. Individuals are, for example, perfectly capable of allowing a fellow team member (whom they dislike) to continue with a course of action that they know to be inappropriate, in the hope that the disliked individual will end up in real trouble that could have been averted by timely intervention. It has been mentioned above that training in team decision making is now a formal requirement in aviation, and it is difficult to see why it should not also have a place in anaesthesia.

WORKING WITH MACHINES AND AUTOMATION

Designing equipment in ways that minimize human error has been dealt with exhaustively,[41–44] yet there remain many differences between known best practice and actual practice. For example, it is clear that using a variety of different, abstract, coded auditory warnings is unwise, yet many intensive therapy units will contain just such a potentially confusing array. A new problem in the design of the human-equipment interface concerns the introduction of computerized and automated machines.

There are a number of characteristics of these devices.[45–48] The first is that information does not need to be displayed to the operator on individual gauges or scales, but may be integrated or fused into a picture presented on a cathode ray tube (CRT) that need not be abstracted or symbolic but may be very representational and pictorial. Thus the operator needs to do less work in order to generate an internal world model since this is effectively generated by the machine. The problem with this is that the display may be so persuasive, and so distanced by the intervening computer (whose software is likely to remain opaque and incomprehensible to the operator) from the sensors that gathered the data, that the operator may have difficulty in troubleshooting the system or even in understanding its normal behaviour. Second, such systems can be designed to be 'intelligent' in preventing certain pre-defined situations from occurring (for example, simply not permitting certain dangerous gas mixtures to be delivered). The difficulty with this is that the operator, relatively ignorant of the system's internal operations, may come to believe that the system will prevent him or her from getting into dangerous situations, thus allowing a situation of 'overtrust' to develop.

Lastly, the computers that drive such systems are so flexible that they may be set up by the operator in many different modes or regimes. A number of aircraft accidents have occurred because pilots believed the computer to be engaged in one mode when actually a quite different one was selected. Clear mode annunciation to prevent these errors of 'mode awareness' is obviously important. As a result of all of these effects, it is said that the most frequently uttered remarks on the flight decks of automated aircraft are either 'I wonder why it's doing that' and 'I've never seen it do that before', and anyone who has used a word processor or video recorder will be able to identify with these difficulties, and will equally realize that adequate training in all of the system's functions is a prerequisite of safe operation.

SYSTEM RESPONSIBILITIES

The balance of responsibility between the individual operator and the general management of the overall system within which he or she works is not presently well resolved. Two conspicuous accidents, the railway accident at Clapham in London and the ferry accident at Zeebrugge in Belgium, have made this issue a matter of public debate.[49,50] There is clearly a responsibility on all individuals to behave in ways that do not jeopardize the safety of those who rely on their expertise, but there must be an equal responsibility that system managers do not expect individual operators to use their human flexibility to compensate for inadequate training, poor equipment, or unreasonable workload and duty hours.[51–55] It is only these managers who are capable of putting into place individual and group training, regular performance monitoring and competence checking, good working practices and procedures, and well designed environments and equipment. It may even be argued that no individual should be held responsible for an incident or accident unless it can be shown that all system factors have been adequately addressed. These issues will remain, of course, matters for judgement in individual cases, but there are two final points that may be made about system responsibility. The first concerns the way in which the system deals with accidents and incidents:[56-59] these should be investigated by an independent agency that does not have any interest either in the individual anaesthetist or in the hospital management. Data from such incidents should be fully encoded and stored in a central database to permit the identification of frequently encountered problems. Furthermore, since many incidents will be known only to the individual anaesthetist, there should be a channel to enable incidents to be reported completely confidentially, again to an independent agency that maintains a central database. It is only by putting in place such feedback loops that system managers may have any confidence that they are able to gain a knowledge of those issues that should be addressed. These procedures have proved very successful in aviation, and could be emulated in many other fields.

The second responsibility of the system is to promote what might be termed a 'safety culture'. Implementing the systems outlined will give an important signal in this regard, but it is even more important to act on the information yielded by them. Everybody who works in a system will appreciate that there will inevitably be compromises between cost and safety, but system managers should try hard to ensure that their decisions do not always appear to be cost driven, and that actions specifically designed to improve safety are given priority. For example, occasions will present themselves when a system manager has a choice between implementing a technological innovation in a way that enables a higher throughput of patients with no reduction in safety or increasing safety with no reduction in throughput. By making safety choices, by keeping staff fully engaged in safety seminars and bulletins, and by ensuring that management attitudes towards safety are substantial rather than superficial, a safety culture may be established that ensures that all staff recognize that minimizing error is a fundamental part of their jobs.

KEY POINTS FOR CLINICAL PRACTICE

- Generating and maintaining an accurate mental or situational model is essential for safe behaviour. Models are based not only on sensed information, but on stored information and expectations. It is important to ensure that situational models do not rely too heavily on expectations in familiar situations, that a good model is created before behaviour is advanced or progressed, and that doubtful models are tested by attempting to disprove them.

- Confirmation bias should be avoided.
- Automated behaviours or skills can be exercized inappropriately in a number of situations, and individuals should attempt to train themselves not to rely too heavily on automated behaviours.
- Conscious intervention or checking that a piece of behaviour is appropriate after it has been selected but before it is executed can help to prevent such errors.
- Drills and procedures are important for safety, and as much as possible of the anaesthetist's task should be proceduralized. The use of explicit anaesthetic plans and checklists are important, and infrequently encountered emergency drills should be practised regularly in a simulated environment in order to ensure behavioural currency in their execution.
- Reasoned behaviours or problem solving should also be practised by generating simulated situations (even if this is carried out only around a desk) in which ill defined and multi-variate problems are tackled, in order to enable the development of problem solving strategies that include gathering, evaluating, and reviewing available information in explicit ways and planning solution paths.
- Performance is affected by acute reactive stress during emergencies, by fatigue, and by life stress. The anaesthetist should be aware of the importance of avoiding such situations, and of how to cope with them when they arise.
- Cognitive and action coping strategies.
- Team decision-making strategies should be developed through simulation and role play to enable the appropriate mix of autocratic and democratic leadership styles to be acquired. The anaesthetist should also train her or himself to make the best use of other operating team members' views and potential solutions to a problem before making his own views or solutions known. Equally he or she should develop techniques for informing other members of the team when he believes that a difficult situation may be developing.
- It is important for the anaesthetist to be alert for design shortcomings in his equipment, and this is especially so as anaesthetic machines become increasingly automated. Particular care should be taken to ensure that the machine's limitations are fully understood, that not too much trust is placed in the machine, and that an awareness of the current operational mode of the machine is maintained.
- Safe clinical practice requires the provision of error reporting systems that are non-punitive and ideally that are operated by a disinterested party. It must be ensured that the information from such systems is utilized in generating system modification, and that a system culture is promoted that causes all operators to appreciate that system safety is brought about by the appropriate actions of all members of that system.

REFERENCES

1. Emergency Care Research Institute: Deaths during general anesthesia. J Health Care Technol 1985; 1: 155–175
2. McDonald J S, Peterson S. Lethal errors in anesthesiology. Anesthesiology 1985; 63: A497
3. Gaba D M. Anesthetic mishaps: breaking the chain of accident evolution. Anesthesiology 1987; 66: 670–676
4. Gaba D M. Human error in anesthetic mishaps. Int Anesthesiol Clin 1989; 27: 137
5. Gaba D M. Human performance issues in anesthesia patient safety. Prob Anesth 1991; 5: 329–350
6. Cooper J B. Toward prevention of anesthetic mishaps. Int Anesthesiol Clin 1984; 22: 167–183
7. Keenan R L. Anesthesia disasters incidence, causes, and preventability. Semin Anesth 1986; 5: 175–179
8. Holland R. Special committee investigating deaths under anaesthesia: report on 745 cases. Med J Aust 1970; 1: 573–593
9. Nagel D C. Human error in aviation operations. In: Wiener E L, Nagel D C, eds. Human factors in aviation. San Diego: Academic Press, 1988; 263
10. Green R. Human error on the flight deck. Phil Trans R Soc Lond 1990; 327: 503–511
11. Goodstein L, Andersen H, Olsen S. Introduction. In: Goodstein K, Andersen H, Olsen S. Tasks, errors and mental models. London: Taylor & Francis, 1988
12. Green R G, Muir H, James M, Gradwell D, Green R L. Human factors for pilots. Aldershot: Ashgate, 1991
13. Einhorn H J, Hogarth R M. Confidence in judgement: persistence of the illusion of validity. Psychol Rev 1978; 85L: 395–416
14. Cook R I, McDonald J S. Cognitive tunnel vision in the operating room, analysis of cases using a frame model. Anesthesiology 1988; 69: A497
15. Woods D, Cook R, Sarter N, McDonald J. Mental models of anesthesia equipment operation: Implications for patient safety. Anesthesiology 1989; 71: A983
16. Sanderson P, Harwood K. The skills, rules and knowledge classification: A discussion of its emergence and nature. In: Goodstein L, Andersen H, Olsen S. Tasks, errors, and mental models. London: Taylor & Francis, 1988
17. Rasmussen J. Skills, rules and knowledge; Signals, signs and symbols, and other distinctions in human performance models. IEEE Trans on Systems, Man, and Cybernetics 1983; SMC-13: 257–266
18. Norman D. Categorization of action slips. Psych-Rev 1981; 88: 1–15
19. Reason J. Human error. Cambridge, UK: Cambridge University Press, 1990
20. Reason J. Modeling the basic error tendencies of human operators. Reliability Engin System Safety 1988; 20: 137–153
21. Rendall-Baker L. Better labels will cut drug errors. Anesthesia Patient Safety Foundation Newsletter 1987; 2: 29
22. DeAnda A, Gaba D. Unplanned incidents during comprehensive anesthesia simulation. Anesth Analg 1990; 71: 77–82
23. DeKeyser V, Woods D. Fixation errors. Failures to revise situation assessment in dynamic and risky systems. In: Columbo A, Bustamante A, eds. Systems reliability assessment. Dordrecht: Kluwer Academic Publishers, 1990
24. Selye H. The stress concept and some of its implications. In: Hamilton V, Warburton D M, eds. Human stress and cognition. Chichester: Wiley, 1979
25. Stokes A, Kite K. Flight stress: stress, fatigue, and performance. Aldershot: Avebury Aviation, 1994
26. Green R. Stress and accidents in aviation. Int J Av Safety 1984: 172–174
27. Toung T J K, Donham R T, Rogers M C. The stress of giving anesthesia on the electrocardiogram of anesthesiologists. Anesthesiology 1984; 61: A465
28. Toung T J K, Donham R T, Rogers M C. The effect of previous medical training on the stress of giving anesthesia. Anesthesiology 1986; 65: A473
29. Johnson L C, Naitoh P. The operational consequences of sleep deprivation and sleep deficit. London, England, North Atlantic Treaty Organization, AGARD Report 1974; #AG-192

30. Woodward D P, Nelson P D. A user-oriented review of the literature on the effects of sleep loss, work-rest schedules, and recovery on performance (Section B), Subcommittee on non-atomic military research and development: human performance and military capability in continuous operations. Washington D.C. The technical Cooperation Program, 1974

31. Bandaret L E, Stokes J W, Francesconi R, Kowal D M, Naitoh P. Artillery teams in simulated sustained combat. Performance and other measures. The 24 hour workday. Proceedings of a symposium on variation in work schedules. Johnson L C, Tepas D I, Colquhoun W P, Colligan M J, eds. Cincinnati, Ohio, U.S. Dept of Health and Human Services. NIOSH Publication 1981; #81–127: 581–604

32. Cooper J B. Do short breaks increase or decrease anesthetic risk? J Clin Anesth 1989; 1: 228–231

33. Dinges D F, Orne M T, Orne E C. Assessing performance upon abrupt awakening from naps during quasi-continuous operations. Behav Res Meth Instru Comput 1985; 17: 37–45

34. Thackray R I, Jones K N, Touchstone R M. Personality and physiological correlates of performance decrement on a monotonous task requiring sustained attention. Br J Soc Psychol 1974; 65: 351–358

35. Joint Aviation Authorities. Flight and duty time limitations and rest requirements. NPA-OPS-4, JAR-OPS Part 1, subpart Q. Hoofddorp: JAA Headquarters, 1993

36. Wegmann H M, Conrad B, Klein K E. Flight, flight duty, and rest times – a comparison between the regulations of different countries. Av Space Env Med 1983; 54: 212–217

37. Lauber J. Cockpit resource management: Background and overview. In: Orlady H W, Foushee H C. Cockpit Resource Management Training, NASA Conference Publication 2455. Washington DC National Aeronautics and Space Administration, 1986

38. Helmreich R L. Cockpit management attitudes. Human Factors 1984; 26: 583–589

39. Helmreich R. Theory underlying CRM training: Psychological issues in flight crew performance and crew coordination. In: Orlady H W, Fouschee H C. Cockpit Resource Management Training, NASA Conference Publication 2455. Washington DC: National Aeronautics and Space Administration, 1986

40. Cooper J B, Newbower R S, London C D, et al. Critical incidents associated with intraoperative exchanges of anesthesia personnel. Anesthesiology 1982; 1: 228–231

41. Mitchell M M. Human Factors in the man-machine interface. The automated anesthesia record and alarm systems. In: Gravenstein J S, Newbower R S, Ream A K, Smith N T S, eds. Boston: Butterworths, 1987; 33–48

42. Cook R, Woods D, McDonald J, Potter S. Human factors standards for operating room equipment: Do they work? Does it matter? Anesthesiology 1989; 71: A335

43. Rasmussen J. Information processing and human-machine interaction: an approach to cognitive engineering. New York: Elsevier Science, 1986

44. Cooper J B, Newbower R, Kitz R. An analysis of major errors and equipment failures in anesthesia management: Considerations for prevention and detection. Anesthesiology 1984; 60: 34–42

45. James M, McClumpha A, Green R, Wilson P, Belyavin A. Pilot attitudes to aircraft automation. In: Human factors on advanced flight decks. London: RAeS, 1991

46. Amalberti R. Cockpit automation: promises and drawbacks. In: Report of the ICAO flight safety regional seminar and workshop. Amsterdam, 1994

47. Billings C. Human-centered automation: a concept and guidelines. NASA Tech Memo 103885. 1991

48. Parasuraman R. Human-computer monitoring. Human Factors 1987; 29: 695–706

49. MV Herald of Free Enterprise: report of court no. 8074. London: HMSO, 1987

50. Hidden A. Investigation into the Clapham Junction railway accident. London: HMSO, 1989

51. Deasy T L. Quality improvement: The gurus and their approaches. Int Anesth Clin 1992; 30: 1–14

52. Schisler J Q. Implementing continuous quality improvement: A private practice's experience. International Anesthesia Clinics 1992; 30: 45–46

53. Duberman S. Quality assurance in the practice of anesthesiology. American Society of Anesthesiologists. Park Ridge Ill. 1986

54. Craig J, Wilson M E. A survey of anaesthetic misadventures. Anaesthesia 1981; 36: 922–936
55. Woods D, O'Brien J, Hanes L. Human factors challenges in process control: The case of nuclear power plants. In: Salvendy G, Handbook of Human Factors. New York: Wiley-Interscience 1987
56. Cook R, Woods D, McDonald J. Human performance in anesthesia: A corpus of cases. CSEL91.003. Cognitive Systems Engineering Laboratory, Department of Industrial and Systems Engineering, Ohio State University 1991
57. Kumar V, Barcellos W A, Mehta M P, Carter J G. An analysis of critical incidents in a teaching department for quality assurance: A survey of mishaps during anaesthesia. Anaesthesia 1988; 43: 879–883
58. Lunn J N, Devlin H B. Lessons from the confidential enquiry into perioperative deaths in three NHS regions. Lancet 1987; 1384–1386
59. Williamson J. Critical incident reporting in anaesthesia. Anaesth Intensive Care 1988; 16: 114–116

2

Record keeping in anaesthesia

W. F. de Mello   A. P. Adams

The anesthetic record is the final arbiter of the manner in which patient care is rendered.[1]

Health care professionals and organizations should adopt the computer-based patient record as the standard for medical and all other records related to patient care.[2]

Improvement in clinical practice, teaching and statistical study must be based on adequate records.[3] On November 30th 1894, or possibly a little earlier, Ernest Amory Codman, a surgical house officer at the Massachusetts General Hospital, created the first known anaesthetic record.[4] His chief, F B Harrington, suggested that records be kept to document the progress of an anaesthetic. These charts gave the following information: name of operation; name of surgeon; exact time the ether administration was begun; amount of ether necessary to anaesthetize the patient; drugs previously administered; the amount of mucus; condition of the heart; charting of the pulse rate and the respiration throughout the entire operation. Codman was a contemporary of the later to be famous neurosurgeon Harvey Cushing and the two young doctors were determined to become good 'etherizers'. Henry Beecher found an anaesthesia chart by Cushing dated July 17th 1895; his chart differed from Codman's and emphasized temperature, pulse and respiration but added in his own handwriting things he thought significant for each case such as vomitus – time and amount, time when the patient came out of the ether, behaviour, the time when the pulse came down, etc.[5] The 'ether charts' which Codman and Cushing devised allowed the anaesthetist and the surgeon to follow the condition of the patient: 'we both became very much more skilled in our jobs . . . particularly due, I think, to the detailed attention which we had to put upon the patient by the careful recording of the pulse rate throughout the operation'. In letters between Codman and Cushing the latter emphasized that careful anaesthesia and record keeping 'was undoubtedly a step toward improvement in what had been a very casual administration of a dangerous drug'.

In 1901 Cushing visited Scipione Riva-Rocci's clinic in Pavia, Italy where beside the bedside of every patient in the Ospedale di S. Matteo was a home-made blood pressure apparatus. Cushing took a model apparatus back with him to the Johns Hopkins Hospital in Baltimore and insisted on its routine use for all his surgical operations.[6] Cushing's efforts marked the beginnings of blood pressure determinations during anaesthesia and his achievements and enormous contributions to the specialty have been documented by Moore,[7] Shephard,[8,9] Vandam[10] and others. Cushing was also responsible for instituting continuous auscultation of cardiac and respiratory rhythm during the entire course of anaesthesia[11,12] and recognized the importance of physician anaesthesia. GW Crile took up the idea of records and was awarded the Cartwright Prize in 1923 of the Alumni Association of the College of Physicians and Surgeons, New York City, for his experiments on blood pressure during surgery: the publication of his monograph was a stimulus to anaesthetists to routinely record the blood pressure during surgical operations.[13] Others such as McKesson,[14] John Lundy,[15] and Ralph Waters in the USA, and Gilbert Brown[16] in Adelaide also popularized the use of record keeping. However, Rovenstine of Madison, Wisconsin, pointed out that statistical reports relating to anaesthesia lacked convincing, statistically reliable evidence.[17] He stressed the importance of uniformity in collecting, correlating and reporting statistics relative to anaesthesia. He recommended the use of tabulating cards and a sorting machine to process the data and in 1933 brought out the first Annual Statistical Report based on these methods.

In 1958 Harry Middleton[18] described a cumulative record system for individual patients and in 1963 Oldham[19] described a new type of combined anaesthetic and operation record. Michael Nosworthy of St Thomas' Hospital in London described the value of anaesthetic records[20] based on a system of punched cards.[21] The cards were 203 mm x 125 mm with 133 holes pre-punched around the perimeter and other parts on the card. Each hole corresponded to a brief printed statement so that the anaesthetist could respond by opening up appropriate holes using a ticket punch. Space was provided for free text entries and a grid for charting the vital signs. The pack of record cards – from a series of anaesthetics – was later sorted using a knitting needle inserted through any given hole. Cards which had been clipped fell from the pack and so could be identified; these could be further sorted according to another parameter (hole) as desired. The Hollerith system of punched cards for sorting data has been used successfully in the US Army for recording anaesthetic and surgical problems.[22,23]

From these modest beginnings has evolved the concept of comprehensive anaesthetic record keeping which forms the basis of safe anaesthetic practice. The modern anaesthetic record contains a lot of data and is no longer of sole interest to anaesthetists but also to other clinicians, nurses, administrators, and occasionally lawyers. In 1978 Seed and Welsh[24] reported the results of a survey by questionnaire of current practice of anaesthetic record keeping by a fairly large sample of consultant anaesthetists who were members of the Association of Anaesthetists (AAGBI) in the British Isles.

It is astonishing that at that particular time some hospitals had no record sheet at all, whereas others used more than one kind of chart: the sole record of the anaesthetic was an entry in the operating theatre register in 3.4% of instances. In 1965 a subcommittee on the standardization of hospital medical records[25] in the UK reported that there were advantages in having essential patient data on a special form for operation and anaesthesia and there was an urgent need for standardization in the design of such forms. Subsequently, the AAGBI suggested a standardized anaesthesia record form for use by anaesthetists working in hospitals where no special provision was made in the patient's notes for the recording of anaesthetic data of either routine or unusual importance.[26] Nevertheless, there still is no national anaesthesia record in the UK.

WHO SHOULD MAKE THE ANAESTHETIC RECORD?

The anaesthetist who sees the patient pre-operatively should initiate the record. The peroperative record should be completed by the anaesthetist administering the anaesthetic or his assistant: 'Our first moments with a patient are packed with visual, auditory and tactile information that determines both the effectiveness and costs of our subsequent care'.[27] The content of most records is text, which is easily transported and stored.

WHY MAKE RECORDS?

Records should be kept for four main reasons: as a tool of patient care; for teaching, audit and research purposes; for administrative purposes; and for medico-legal reasons.

A tool of patient care

The anaesthetic record embraces details from the pre-operative to the postoperative period. After the pre-operative visit, the record should contain a summary which includes patient identification, surgical details and nature of the proposed surgery, past medical history, previous anaesthetics, addiction, medication, allergies, family history, review of systems, clinical findings with emphasis to the surgery/anaesthetic proposed, record of the vital signs, weight, results of investigations, details optimizing the patient's medical status (premedication, instructions for restrictions of food and fluid intake, deep vein thrombosis and antibiotic prophylaxis, etc.). This serves as an *aide memoire* during the course of the anaesthetic.

The intraoperative record contains information such as anaesthetic and monitoring equipment checks, date, time and location of the operation, monitoring, induction, airway management, anaesthetic technique, drugs and interventions, fluid fluxes, complications or critical incidents and, of course, a record of vital signs and other monitored variables. The act of recording information by hand on the chart forces the anaesthetist to be aware of the time-course and detail of anaesthetic events[28] because he or she must look at the monitors and process the information in the brain before committing it to paper. Because the monitored variables are plotted on a grid, the record demonstrates the *trend*, with respect to time, that allows identification of change that could not be obtained from just observing individual values from the monitor. It also helps demonstrate the relationship between a drug administration, therapeutic intervention, or both, and the physiological response. However, it is possible to create a scenario in which the anaesthetist relies on an automatically constructed recorded trend without pausing to investigate its cause and likely transient nature and acts inappropriately, hence the need for caution against overdependence on machine-generated trends.[29]

The postoperative record should contain details of observations and interventions required: oxygen therapy, fluid administration, prescription of analgesia, antiemetics, antibiotics, deep vein thrombosis prophylaxis and other drugs, expected or anticipated problems and their management, and any immediate or long term implications for future anaesthetics or general health. The whole record allows subsequent anaesthetics to be planned accordingly.

Following the Access to Health Records Act 1990, patients are now entitled to inspect their own records and have inaccurate entries corrected.[30] Doctors and nurses looking after the patient are entitled to perusal of medical records as is the Health Authority to ensure its duty of care in the defence of litigation and audit. Burnum[31] suggested that US physicians are now deliberately misrecording patient data to avoid litigation, and this alarming notion is supported by a study of anaesthetists who showed striking reluctance to record extreme blood pressure values:[32] none of four systolic readings above 205 mmHg or of 33 diastolic readings above 110 mmHg appeared in the notes, even though they were documented by a carefully calibrated machine. The authors suggest that 'the paucity of extreme values in the handwritten record may be an unconscious defensive strategy'.

Teaching, audit and research purposes

The use of personal medical records for research purposes has been threatened by the recent guidelines from the Department of Health, the British Medical Association and the European Commission.[33] It is useful to peruse anaesthetic records not only as an educational exercise but also as a source of audit and for research purposes. Examining records of cases where critical incidents/mortality have occurred can be a useful educational tool. A comprehensive system comprising a database has been developed to study multiple pre-operative patient factors and intraoperative anaesthetic variables with the data linked, describing the casemix and process of care, to several measures of outcome in a large group of patients.[34] Analysis of this database has been useful for research of adverse outcome following anaesthesia, the experience profiles of trainee anaesthetists and the administrative management of the anaesthetics department. Audit of the use of monitors, completeness of records, etc. are an essential part of a quality assurance and peer-review programme. Research benefits can include evaluation of new techniques, drugs, equipment, interventions, etc.

Lilleywhite and Ward[35] candidly report on the accuracy of an anaesthetic computer-based audit system in their hospital. Their results are cause for concern: only half of the notes of patients anaesthetised 4 months previously could be found, and in 40% of these there was no anaesthetic chart. The medico-legal implications in the event of a mishap are evident. They conclude that the overall accuracy of their computerized audit system was between 33 and 52% – and make a plea for auditing the audit system. Sometimes it is forgotten that a computer is not a prerequisite for medical audit. However, computers can make the process cost-effective if used properly and Fisher has explained the advantages and the pitfalls of using computers for audit.[36]

Administrative purposes

The record can help the clinical director in aspects of practice such as manpower allocation, quality of care and quality assurance, patient outcome, anaesthetic practice patterns, use of drugs and equipment, budgetary planning, etc. Departmental statistics can be completed on a weekly, monthly or even an annual basis. It is possible to monitor crude output of the number of anaesthetics administered, anaesthesia person hours, trainee supervision ratios, regional versus general anaesthesia ratios, workload trends in specialty areas, emergency/elective case ratios, drug and agent usage, and even departmental expenditure per anaesthetic or per hour.[37] The hospital administrator or theatre manager can use the details from the anaesthetic record to ensure efficient and cost effective use of staff, equipment and supplies. In these days of financial and budgetary constraints the record can form the basis of reimbursement for anaesthetic services although this is not as widespread in the United Kingdom as in North America.

Medico-legal purposes

Ideally, the anaesthetic record should be an accurate and complete synopsis of what happened during the course of the anaesthetic. There should be sufficient detail to explain peroperative complications or events. It is a paradox that at times of emergency, record keeping is at its poorest; in this instance automated anaesthetic record keepers (AARKs) are valuable. Although there is no statute which requires an anaesthetist to keep a record of an anaesthetic administered, there is a common law requirement for such records to be kept under the Bolam principle.[38] Since clinical practice that does not move with the times is difficult to defend, it is clear that entries in anaesthetic records should be comprehensive, accurate and legible. Besides the court, other interested parties such as the coroner, the police, insurance companies and employers may have the right to patient records in certain circumstances.[39] Insurers have to settle cases, often at considerable expense, where the doctor's recollection of his or her clinical management had been perfectly correct but the clinical records have not confirmed this. Counsel have advised in a number of cases that a court, sympathetic to a damaged patient, will be eager to argue that poor records are indicative of slipshod treatment and care. Insurers such as the Medical Defence Organizations are forever advising their members to make adequate and legible contemporaneous notes which should be signed and dated.[40] If a note of an important event cannot be made at the time of the event, it should be detailed in the notes as soon as possible thereafter. The doctor should also spell out his name in block letters and it is sensible also to write down the time the note was made.

WHAT SHOULD THE ANAESTHETIC RECORD CONTAIN?

It makes little sense to collect, store and distribute data without ensuring its quality. The criteria for an anaesthetic record has been summarized:[41]

- To be accurate, i.e. a minimum of missing or erroneous data and artefact free
- Be complete
- Be legible and interpretable
- Be in real time
- Be immediately available
- Allow pattern recognition and trend detection related to real time
- Allow assessment of response to therapeutic interventions
- Improve cost-effectiveness of patient care.

Although there have been attempts to create a comprehensive anaesthetic record by bodies such as the American Society of Anesthesiologists (ASA), the Royal College of Surgeons of England[42] and the Faculty of Anaesthetists of the Royal Australian College of Surgeons (now the Australian and New Zealand College of Anaesthetists)[43] there is still considerable debate as to what information should be contained in such a document. It is impossible to design a brief record template to cater for all types of patients/procedures/anaesthetic techniques etc., but some of the minimal data that should be incorporated is shown in Table 2.1.

Table 2.1   Information to be noted on an anaesthetic record. Suggestions as to a reasonable content. RCA = Royal College of Anaesthetists. NCEPOD = National Confidential Enquiry into Peri-operative Deaths. Form to be signed and dated.

Pre-operative information
  PATIENT IDENTITY
    Patient name/number
    Gender
    Date of birth
  ASSESSMENT
    Assessor
    Where assessed
    ASA status ± comment
    Date of assessment
    Weight (kg), Height (m)
    Basic vital signs (BP, HR)
    Previous GAs and family history
    Addiction (tobacco, alcohol, drugs, etc.)
    Potential airway problems
    Problems with venous access
    Prostheses
    Investigations
      (i) allergies
      (ii) relevant medication
      (iii) abnormalities to be recorded

  URGENCY
    As per National Critical Incident study

Peroperative Information

  CHECKS
    Nil by mouth; consent; effect of premedication

  PLACE & TIME
    Place
    Date
    Start Time
    End Time

  PERSONNEL
    Anaesthetist 1
    Anaesthetist 2
    Operating Surgeon
    Qualified assistant present
    Note: The RCA and CEPOD recommend that non-consultants must be able to obtain consultant advice at all times. It may be local policy to record the supervising consultant.

  OPERATION PERFORMED

  APPARATUS
    Check performed
      Anaesthetic room
      Operating theatre

  VITAL SIGNS RECORDING/ CHARTING

  DRUGS & FLUIDS
    Time & route
    Injection site
    Dose, concentration & volume
    Additives

  AIRWAY
    Route
    Ventilation mode
    System used
    Airway type, size, cuff, shape
    Gas/vapour – flow/concentration
    Special procedures
    Difficulty

  REGIONAL ANAESTHESIA
    Consent obtained
    Block performed
    Type
    Technique
    Entry site
    Needle used
    Aid to location
    Catheter y/n

  PATIENT POSITION

Postoperative Instructions
    Oxygen instructions
    Drugs & doses
    Fluids
    Special airway instructions

Untoward events
    Abnormalities
    Critical incidents
    Complications
      Preop – Perop – Postop
      Context – Cause – Effect

  HAZARD FLAGS
    Warnings for future care

WHEN SHOULD THE RECORDS BE CREATED?

Ideally the anaesthetic record should be created in real time. However, in the majority of cases where records are manually created, the entries are often recorded retrospectively. Entries are often difficult or impossible to make during critical phases such as the induction or emergence from anaesthesia or during emergencies. The gaps in recording are obvious and even when an attempt is made to fill in the gaps later these entries are often selective, rounded up, or even ignored. This is one of the benefits of AARKs. For medico-legal purposes it is sufficient to show evidence that all information is recorded as soon as possible after the event and late entries signed and dated. The frequency of recording vital signs is also an area of controversy. For example, should pulse, blood pressure, etc., be noted every five minutes? It has been argued that the frequency of vital sign recording should reflect the speed and variation in the parameters themselves; however, a vital sign cannot be said to remain unchanged unless measured.

HOW SHOULD THE ANAESTHETIC RECORD BE KEPT?

It is easy to list the information that ought to be recorded on an anaesthetic chart (Table 2.1), but it is more difficult to decide how a legible record should be presented in a manner that allows the anaesthetist the facility to interpret the information recorded. It must allow the relationship between vital signs and iatrogenic interventions to be displayed, so that the trend plotting and its interpretation will allow appropriate action to be initiated. Although the majority of today's records are created manually, current technology is sophisticated enough to partially or fully automate such records. The handwritten record has the advantage of being widely accepted, portable, inexpensive, easy to use, and allows subjective descriptions or notations to be added. The disadvantages include the time-consuming effort of creating a record usually at the cost of patient surveillance, accuracy, legibility, completeness, difficulty in retrieving information and the potential for loss. Only records that are legible can be considered as a useful means of communication: only automation can consistently improve legibility. During the induction of anaesthesia, vital signs fluctuate significantly. However, only a few of these changes are likely to be recorded because the anaesthetist is fully occupied with life-support measures; attending to the record would be an inappropriate distraction from essential medical observation and care. Once the operation is underway and the patient is stable, the anaesthetist tries to reconstruct the record of the preceding events from memory: inaccuracies and omissions are inevitable.[44] Several studies have confirmed that entries by the anaesthetist are untimely during periods of induction, emergence or during critical incidents. Furthermore, entries made in retrospect are often inaccurate, and the bias in determining what entries are to be entered or ignored or rounded up to a more acceptable value.[45,46] How often the record should be updated during the course of an anaesthetic is a matter of debate. Most choose the entirely arbitrary time of 5 minutes. This may satisfy the needs of an uneventful routine minor surgical case, but would this also be true for complex cases where physiological trespass is marked from either the patient's physical status, surgery being performed or the type of anaesthesia being administered?

WHERE SHOULD THE ANAESTHETIC RECORD BE STORED AFTER ITS COMPLETION?

Obviously, a copy should go into the patient's notes. If there are any anaesthetic details that need to be brought to the attention of the patient's general practitioner (such as anaphylaxis, difficult intubation, malignant hyperpyrexia, etc.) then either a summary or a copy of the record should be sent. There is an obvious need for maintaining the confidentiality of medical information and, with the increasing use of computers and information technology in health care, steps must be taken to prevent a breach in security by hackers. Information from the anaesthetic record may be held by the operating theatre administrators, the anaesthetic department, research groups, by individual anaesthetists to compile their log books, and by other health care workers. It must be remembered that medical records are the property of the hospital, but the information contained in them is the property of the patient. The consultant is the custodian of that information and his or her permission should be sought before any disclosure is made. Breach of this confidentiality can only be made with the consent of the patient or by order of the courts. Records should be retained for 8 years or if involving obstetric cases for 25 years.[47]

THE FUTURE

The disadvantages of paper-based systems are described by Wyatt.[48] They may be improved in four ways: change their contents, change their format, store them differently, and change their form. Anaesthetists are most interested in the format aspect because speed in completing entries can be facilitated by using, for example, a pre-printed form clearly laid out where items are either circled or ticked and the need for free handwritten narrative reduced to a minimum. The future lies in the increasing use of information technology in health care. Thrush[46] concluded from a study comparing 13 handwritten with 13 computer-generated anaesthesia records that observer bias, missed readings and errors of memory which affect manual records may cause significant inaccuracy and may be avoided by using automated anaesthesia records generated by information management systems. Substantial differences in vital signs data are often noted when values recorded automatically are compared with values recorded manually by an anaesthetist using the same monitors. In the case of systolic blood pressure, for example, 32% of readings differed by a mean of more than 10 mmHg (range 74 to 95 mmHg).[49] Some of the characteristics of AARKs are summarized in Table 2.2 and their advantages and disadvantages listed in Table 2.3. These include the acquisition, recording and charting of monitored variables and the quick inputting of text and numerical information in a safe, reproducible and retrievable form. Introduction has been slow because of the costs of introducing such systems and integrating it with other devices such as the monitors, its reluctant acceptance by anaesthetists who view the machine-user interface as unfriendly, the fear of a true presentation of anaesthetic events, the difficulty in making notations easily, and the fear of artefacts.

Table 2.2   Characteristics of automated anaesthesia record-keeping systems[41]

- Technically feasible
- Mixed automatic and manual input
- Neat legible output
- Appear more accurate
- Useful for clinical audit
- Useful for training
- User/computer interface still a problem

Table 2.3   Advantages and disadvantages of automated anaesthesia record-keeping systems.

ADVANTAGES
- Improves quality
- Permits complete accuracy and better legibility
- Is easier to archive the information
- Improves access to medical records from the archives
- Facilitates research
- Allows prospective multicentric or comparative studies
- Improves vigilance?
- Facilitates billing of patients

DISADVANTAGES
- Cost
- Not user friendly
- Reduced vigilance?
- Problem of artefacts
- Does not necessarily improve patient care
- Does not reduce the anaesthetist's workload
- Technological limitations

However, the entry frequency is enhanced by AARKs and it is quite possible to retain high-resolution data during periods of interest, and low-resolution data during routine ones. AARKs can either print the record simultaneously or store it on tapes/disks and print later. The latter offers a greater facility of examining details of epochs which is not possible with either written or simultaneous automated systems. In order to ensure completeness of AARK records, reminders in the form of messages, checklists or automated prompts can be incorporated. The legibility of the record is important and, not surprisingly, the automated one is superior to that handwritten.[50] Not only should the record be legible so as to portray the course of the anaesthetic but also in its secondary aim of satisfying the medico-legal requirements. The prime disadvantage of automated records is medico-legal. Eichhorn[29] quotes Morris, a noted defence attorney in the US, who frankly stated 'I desperately need it if it says what I want to say; but if not, I'm not sure I want it in the courtroom'. Because handwritten entries are not being made by the anaesthetist when AARK systems are used, there is concern that lack of vigilance of physiological trends, or awareness of monitored variables may be a problem[51] and could result in sub-optimal care. The solution lies in proper training of trainees. AARKs faithfully display what is displayed on the monitor: artefacts are thus not necessarily automatically rejected. Between 0.1 and 6% of data captured by automated systems has been shown to be artefactual depending on the kind of variable measured[52] but encouragingly the incidence is decreasing with modern technology. The possibility that the automated device will indiscriminately record data whether valid or invalid and that the invalid data, the artefacts, might be subsequently interpreted as valid is of major concern to anaesthetists. It should be possible for the anaesthetist to add an initialled handwritten comment to the record in the event of an artefact. The anaesthetist wishes to keep control over what appears on the record with the aim of minimizing the chance of any possible litigation. If important data has been suppressed at will by the anaesthetist, and this comes to light during a law suit, all anaesthetists and all their records become vulnerable. A jury is more likely to believe the clinician who candidly presents all data, good and bad, than one who filters and smooths the data.[44]

It would seem logical that if the time spent in recording data was reduced by the use of AARKs then this saving in time could be put to better use in improving patient care. However, critics point to the possibility of a reduction in the anaesthetist's awareness of monitored data and the lack of evidence to support improved patient care. AARKs reduce the tedium of filling in the anaesthetic record, but there is still considerable information that may have to be entered such as details of the patient, the procedure, drugs administered, notations of events expected and unexpected, etc. In one time and motion study, partial automation did not reduce documentation time when compared to conventional methods.[53] However, another study did show a considerable saving of time with automation:[54] total anaesthesia time was about 34 minutes in two comparable groups of patients. In the manual records group charting took 13.3 minutes on average whilst in the automated group it only occupied 4.7 minutes. Moreover, the amount of recorded information was six-fold higher in the automated group and surprisingly the number of free text entries by the anaesthetist was also increased in this group.

The standard data entry device is commonly the 'Qwerty' keyboard, although other devices such as a 'mouse', soft key, bar code readers,[55] voice recognition systems,[56] and touch screens have also been tried. The need for manual notation of information remains a hindrance to smooth automation of anaesthetic records. Another problem is the compatibility of the monitoring equipment with the computer and the means of data storage. Once equipment has been standardized and a common data set and national and international drug codes agreed upon, automation and comparison across national borders is facilitated. The need for rejecting spurious data automatically, and the availability of 'knowledge based' software, that can provide intelligent suggestions to complement the clinical decisions of the anaesthetist, must be the way forward.

With the eventual establishment of a medical information highway, and assuming the practical problems that currently prevent a super-efficient electronic communication network are solved, there is still a need to create a single medical language such as the Read Codes and the Terms project.[57] Possibly in the near future each patient will carry his or her own 'smart card' that will either store all personal health data or allow the information to be accessed, by a health worker with the appropriate password, from a central database. In Europe, it is proposed that the health record be comprehensive and medicolegally accepted across clinical domains, hold all data types, and be automatically translated between languages.[58] The application of advanced information technology to patient records means that there will be an expanding database that could be readily available to all health care providers. This raises ethical issues such as status of the electronic record, data ownership, data liability, informed consent to use, retrieval, security and access. These ethical problems need to be addressed in a co-ordinated international fashion and receive appropriate legal expression in the relevant countries and be incorporated into appropriate codes of ethics.[59]

The Royal College of Anaesthetists' Quality of Practice Committee has set up a subcommittee (1994/5) to advise the College on what is needed to be recorded on the anaesthetic record (Table 2.1 is a draft of likely proposals): it was not felt necessary to distinguish between manually and electronically collected data, nor was there a brief to design a universal record. It may be easier to create a unique format for sub-specialist groups such as acute and chronic pain, obstetrics, day case surgery, cardiac and neuro-anaesthesia etc. The need to comply with legislation regarding product liability[60] means that anaesthetists should record details of all devices used on their patients. Input from SCATA (Society for Computing and Technology in Anaesthesia) was valuable and a draft field set for the anaesthetic record has now been produced. This data considers the minimum data required regarding pre-operative information, peroperative information, and postoperative information. A number of commercial automated systems have now become available: these vary in ease of use and acceptance and need to be tried extensively before commitment to high cost purchase.[61]

REFERENCES

1. Feldman J M. The Anesthetic Record. In: Kirby R R (ed) Clinical Anesthesia Practice. W. B. Saunders: London 1994: pp 20–30
2. Summary. In: Dick R S, Steen E B (eds) The Computer-based Patient Record: an essential technology for healthcare. National Academy Press: Washington DC, 1991: p 6.
3. Waters R M, Rovenstine E A, Lundy J S et al. Subcommittee on Anesthesia of Division of Medical Sciences, National Research Council. Fundamentals of Anesthesia: an outline. Second edn. American Medical Association Press, Chicago, 1944: pp 3–8
4. Beecher H K. The first anesthesia records (Codman, Cushing). Surg Gynecol Obstet 1940; 71: 689–693
5. Keys T E. The History of Surgical Anesthesia. Dover Publications, New York, 1963: p 87
6. Hirsch N, Smith G. Harvey Cushing: his contribution to anesthesia. Anesth Analg 1986; 65: 288–293
7. Moore F D. Harvey Cushing: general surgeon, biologist, professor. J Neurosurg 1969; 31: 262–270
8. Shephard D A E. Harvey Cushing and anaesthesia. Can Anaes Soc J. 1965; 12: 832–42
9. Shephard D A E. Cushing's contribution to anesthesia: two comments. Anesth Analg 1968; 65: 1251–1252
10. Vandam L D. Cushing's contribution to anesthesia: two comments. Anesth Analg 1968; 65: 1249–1251
11. Cushing H W. Some principles of cerebral surgery. JAMA 1909; 532: 184–192
12. Fulton J F. Harvey Cushing – a biography. Thomas, Springfield Illinois, 1946: p 218
13. Crile G W. Blood-pressure in surgery. Lippincott, Philadelphia, 1903.
14. McKesson E I. Blood pressure in general anesthesia. Am J Surg Anesth Suppl 1916; 30: 2–5
15. Lundy J S. Keeping anesthetic records and what they show. Am J Surg (Quart Suppl Anesth and Analg) 1924; 38: 16–25
16. Brown G. Notes on 300 cases of general anaesthesia combined with narcotics. Lancet 1911; i: 1005–1006
17. Rovenstine E A. A method of combining anesthetic and surgical records for statistical purposes. Anesth Analg 1934; 13: 122–128
18. Middleton H. A cumulative anaesthesia record system. Anaesthesia 1958; 13: 337
19. Oldham K W. Anaesthetic and operation records. A description of a new type of combined form. Anaesthesia 1963; 18: 213–216
20. Nosworthy M D. The value of anaesthetic records. St Thomas' Hospital Reports 1937; 2: 54–66
21. Nosworthy M D. Method of keeping anaesthetic records and assessing results. Br J Anaesth 1943; 18: 160–179
22. Wangeman C P, Martin S J. The recording of surgical and anesthetic data in two Army general hospitals. Anesthesiology 1945; 6: 64–80
23. Fundamentals of Anesthesia. An outline. Subcommittee on Anesthesia of Division of Medical Sciences, National Research Council. American Medical Association Press, Chicago, 1944: pp 1–8
24. Seed R F, Welsh E A. Anaesthetic records in Great Britain and Ireland. Anaesthesia 1976; 31: 1199–1210

25. STANDING MEDICAL ADVISORY COMMITTEE. The Standardization of Hospital Medical Records. Her Majesty's Stationary Office, London, 1965: p 26
26. Minutes of Association of Anaesthetists' Sub-Committee set up to consider anaesthetic records. Chairman: Professor W W Mushin, 1965
27. Clark D A. Verbal uncertainty expressions: a critical review of two decades of research. Curr Psychol Res Rev 1990; 9: 203–235
28. Noel T A. Computerized anesthesia records may be dangerous. Anesthesiology 1986; 64: 300
29. Eichhorn J H. Disadvantages of automated anesthesia records. In: Gravenstein J S, Holzer J F (eds) Safety and Cost Containment in Anesthesia. Butterworths, London, 1988: pp 223–231
30. Access to Health Records Act 1990: a guide for the NHS. UK Government Health Department, 1990
31. Burnum J F. The mis-information era: the fall of the medical record. Ann Intern Med 1989; 110: 482–484
32. Cook R I, McDonald J D, Nunziata E. Differences between handwritten and automatic blood pressure records. Anesthesiology 1989; 71: 385–390
33. Wald N, Law M, Meade T et al. Use of personal medical records for research purposes. Br Med J 1994; 309: 1422–1424
34. Rose D K, Cohen M M, Wigglesworth D F, Yee D A. Development of a computerized database for the study of anaesthesia care. Can J Anaesth 1992; 39: 716–723
35. Lilleywhite N, Ward P. Accuracy of a computer-based anaesthetic audit system. Anaesthesia 1993; 48: 885–886
36. Fisher M F. Computers and medical audit. In: Secker-Walker J (ed) Quality and Safety in Anaesthesia. BMJ Publishing Group, London, pp 129–153
37. Holland R. The scope for computerisation in anaesthesia. Anaesth Intens Care 1982; 10: 185–187
38. Address to the jury in the case of *Bolam v Friern Hospital Management Committee* 1957: 2 All ER 118 at 122
39. Powers M J. Record keeping in anaesthesia: what the law requires. Br J Anaesth 1994; 73: 22–24
40. Doherty R. Who needs medical records? The Clinician in Management 1993; 2(5): 2–3
41. Clutton-Brock T H. Does automatic record keeping really help? In: Hutton P (ed) Awareness in anaesthesia and awareness of current issues. Oxford Clinical Communications, Oxford, 1993: p 16
42. Clinical Audit and Quality Assurance Committee. Guidelines for clinicians on medical records and notes. Royal College of Surgeons of England: London, 1990
43. The Anaesthetic Record. Faculty of Anaesthetists, Royal Australasian College of Surgeons Bulletin 1984; 4: 34–36
44. Whitcher C. Advantages of automated record keeping. In: Gravenstein J S, Holzer J F (eds) Safety and Cost Containment in Anesthesia. Butterworths, London, 1988: pp 207–221
45. Galletly D C, Rowe W L, Henderson R S. The anesthetic record: A confidential survey on data omission or modification. Anaesth Intens Care 1991; 19: 74–78
46. Thrush D N. Are automated anesthesia records better? J Clin Anesth 1992; 4: 386–389
47. The Department of Health. Health services management – preservation, retention and destruction of records. Health Publications Unit HC, Heywood, (89) p 20
48. Wyatt J C. Clinical data systems Part 1: Data and medical records. Lancet 1944; 344: 1543–1547
49. Paulus D A, van der Aa J J, McLaughlin G, et al. A semiautomated anesthesia record keeper: a clinical evaluation, abstracted. J Clin Monit 1985; 1: 286–287
50. Gravenstein J S. The uses of the anesthesia record. J Clin Monit 1989; 5: 256–65
51. Edsall D W. Analysis and frequency of artifacts generated by anesthesia information management systems. Anesthesiology 1990; 73: A481
52. Stanley T E, Smith L R, White W D et al. Incidence of vital sign artifact in automated anesthesia records. Anesthesiology 1990; 73: A483
53. Osswald P M, Winter D, Hartung H J, Gasteiger P. NAPROS: A semiautomatic user-friendly anaesthetic record system. Int J Clin Mon Comp 1987; 4: 231–236

54. Edsall D W, Deshane P, Giles C et al. Computerized patient anesthesia records: less time and better quality than manually produced anesthesia records. J Clin Anesth 1993; 5: 275–283

55. Block F E, Burton L W, Rafal M D et al. Two computer-based anesthetic monitors: the Duke automatic monitoring equipment (DAME) system and the microdame. J Clin Monit 1985; 1: 30–51

56. Smith N T, Brien R A, Pettus D C et al. Recognition accuracy with a voice-recognition system designed for anesthesia record keeping. J Clin Monit 1990; 6: 299–306

57. Information Management Group NHS CCC. Read Codes and the Terms Project: a brief guide. 1994. NHS Center for Coding and Classification, Woodgate, Loughborough, LE112TG, England, UK

58. Kalra D. Electronic health record: the European scene. Br Med J 1994; 309: 1358–1361

59. Kluge E H. Advanced patient records: some ethical and legal considerations touching medical information space. Methods of Information in Medicine 1993; 32(2): 95–103

60. Adams A P. Safety in Anaesthetic Practice. In: Atkinson R S, Adams A P (eds) Recent Advances in Anaesthesia & Analgesia - 17. Churchill Livingstone: London, 1992; 1–24

61. Kenny G N C (ed) Automated anaesthetic records. Baillière's Clinical Anaesthesiology. International Practice and Research. 1990; 4(1): 1–252

3

Anaesthesia for minimally invasive abdominal surgery

J. F. Brichant

Although laparoscopy was first described at the beginning of the century,[1] therapeutic laparoscopic surgical procedures have only recently become well established being somewhat ignored until the late 1960s. In 1967, Steptoe[2] described a laparoscopic technique for use in simple pelvic procedures (tubal ligation, ovarian cystectomies, etc.). This technique, which became rapidly popular among gynaecologists, required a pneumoperitoneum and steep head-down position with potential haemodynamic and respiratory consequences. However, these problems were found to be of little significance during short gynaecological procedures performed on young and healthy patients. In the late 1980s, laparoscopic cholecystectomy was described and has become well established.[3–6] With the demonstration that laparoscopic cholecystectomy can be performed safely, several other new intra-abdominal laparoscopic techniques have been described for gastrointestinal and urological surgery.[7] These new techniques are usually prolonged, leading to longer intraperitoneal gas insufflation. They also require significant changes in patient position. In addition, these techniques might be applied to older patients who may have known or latent coexisting cardiac and/or pulmonary disease. Hence, the changes of haemodynamic and respiratory function might be of greater significance. A thorough knowledge of the pathophysiologic changes associated with laparoscopy are of extreme importance for the anaesthetist in charge of patients undergoing laparoscopic surgery. In the light of these changes, he/she will have to weigh up the potential benefits and complications for each patient.

RESPIRATORY CHANGES ASSOCIATED WITH LAPAROSCOPY

Laparoscopy alters respiration; the occurrence of hypercapnia during laparoscopy has been reported from the onset of this technique.[8–10] The increase in $Paco_2$ varies with patient's characteristics, duration of pneumoperitoneum, insufflated gas and anaesthetic technique. Moderate hypoxaemia has also been reported, although it is usually not of clinical significance, except in patients with respiratory, cardiovascular disease or other concomitant disease.[10,11]

Ventilatory changes associated with laparoscopy might be related to changes in patient position and/or to intraperitoneal insufflation of gas and the ensuing increased intra-abdominal pressure.

Ventilatory effects of changes in patient position

The type of surgery will determine patient posture during laparoscopy. The head-down position (Trendelenburg) is used for pelvic and sub-mesocolic surgery, whereas the head-up tilt is used for upper abdominal surgery. These positions contribute to alterations of gas exchange and/or respiratory mechanics.

Alteration of gas exchange

General anaesthesia alters ventilation and perfusion distribution.[12] These alterations differ with patient posture as follows: in the supine posture, ventilation and perfusion are both decreased in the bases of the lung during general anaesthesia while, in the apices of the lung, ventilation is increased and perfusion is not altered; in the sitting position, general anaesthesia increases ventilation and decreases perfusion at the bottom of the lungs whereas, in the top of the lungs, ventilation is slightly decreased and perfusion is almost abolished. Hence, $\dot{V}A/Q$ matching would be better in the sitting than in the supine position in normal subjects under general anaesthesia. This suggests that during general anaesthesia the head-up position would improve $\dot{V}A/Q$ matching, decreasing shunt and physiological dead space. This is in agreement with a recent study suggesting that alveolar dead space is not affected by the steepness of the head-up position.[13]

There are no reports so far about the effects of the head-down position on the distribution of ventilation and pulmonary blood flow. In patients under epidural or local anaesthesia, physiological dead space is unaltered by a head-down tilt; these data suggest that the head-down position minimally alters gas exchange in healthy subjects.[14,15]

Alteration of the mechanics of respiration

The Trendelenburg position might significantly impair respiratory mechanics as it increases the pressure of the abdominal content on the diaphragm. The ensuing cephalad shift of the diaphragm decreases functional residual capacity (FRC), total lung volume and pulmonary compliance. Such changes would favour the development of pulmonary complications such as atelectasis. In fact, these changes are generally moderate.[16] Likewise, currently available data suggest that respiratory mechanics is minimally affected by the head-up position. However, in obese or respiratory disabled patients, respiratory alteration associated with changes in patient posture might be more significant.

Respiratory changes associated with intra-abdominal insufflation of gas

Intraperitoneal insufflation of gas is associated with gas diffusion from the peritoneal cavity and an alteration of gas exchange.[17] Gas insufflation in the peritoneal cavity results in absorption of gas from the peritoneal cavity. Carbon dioxide (CO_2), the gas most often used for laparoscopy, is a highly diffusible gas and thus expected to be captured through the peritoneum.[17] As CO_2 is carried by systemic and portal veins to the pulmonary circulation via the right heart this would result in increased pulmonary CO_2 excretion ($\dot{V}CO_2$) and high $PaCO_2$ if mechanical ventilation is maintained constant. Evidence to suggest absorption of CO_2 from the peritoneal cavity is confirmed by the increased $PaCO_2$ and $\dot{V}CO_2$ observed where CO_2 is used as insufflation gas, contrasting with the constant $PaCO_2$ reported when nitrous oxide (N_2O) is the insufflating gas.[14,18,19] $\dot{V}CO_2$ increases progressively and plateaus after approximately 20 min at 125% of the initial value.[20-22] However, several reports failed to find an increased $\dot{V}CO_2$ during laparoscopy.[15]

From theoretical computations, one would expect larger increases in $\dot{V}CO_2$ and $PaCO_2$. The limited increase actually observed can be explained by the impaired peritoneal perfusion (see haemodynamic changes) and the buffering capacity of the blood. Once in the blood, a large amount of CO_2 is rapidly hydrated to carbonic acid (H_2CO_3) and subsequently ionized to hydrogen (H^+) and bicarbonate (HCO_3^-) ions. A small amount of CO_2 is metabolized to carbonic compounds and transported by haemoglobin.

Another consequence of abdominal cavity distension is a cephalad shift of the diaphragm. The ensuing $\dot{V}A/Q$ mismatching results in an increased physiological dead space, as shown by the increased arterial to alveolar gradient for partial pressure of carbon dioxide [$(a-A)DCO_2$].[8,15,23,24] This increased physiological dead space results in an increased $PaCO_2$ if minute ventilation is maintained constant. Another possible mechanism for increased $(a-A)DCO_2$ is the reduced cardiac output associated with laparoscopy. This increase in $(a-A)DCO_2$ is usually moderate in healthy patients; several studies failed to find an increased $(a-A)DCO_2$ during laparoscopy.[21,22] Increases $(a-A)DCO_2$ are larger in ASA II and III patients than in healthy patients.[24,25]

Influence of anaesthesia

Laparoscopic surgery has been performed under local anaesthesia, regional anaesthesia, general anaesthesia with spontaneous breathing and under general anaesthesia with controlled ventilation. In patients undergoing laparoscopy under local or regional anaesthesia, $PaCO_2$ is unaltered by intraperitoneal insufflation of gas.[14,15] However, minute ventilation is increased, mainly by an increased frequency of breathing, in order to minimize the increase in respiratory work. The constant $Paco_2$ is explained by the absence of ventilatory depressant effect associated with local anaesthetics. In spontaneously breathing patients under general anaesthesia, intraperitoneal insufflation of CO_2 increases minute ventilation. However, this hyperventilation is not large enough to prevent CO_2 from increasing. Rises in $Paco_2$ up to 8.1 ±1.5 kPa (60.8 ± 10.9 mmHg) had been reported in the 1970s.[9] This is related to the ventilatory depressant effect of the general anaesthetic agents that blunt the ventilatory response to hypercapnia and to loading (i.e. increased intra-abdominal pressure).

In short procedures it is unlikely that major hypercapnia will occur. Indeed, CO_2 rises progressively after the start of the gas insufflation and will plateau after 15–25 minutes.[20–22] Last but not least, cardiac and/or respiratory disabled patients will manifest larger respiratory alteration than healthy patients.[24,25] When patients are ventilated mechanically at a constant minute volume, $Paco_2$ increases.[8,19,20]

Postoperative respiratory alterations

Upper abdominal surgery results in postoperative pulmonary alterations: restrictive pulmonary impairment, decreased FRC and diaphragmatic dysfunction. The effects of laparoscopy and laparotomy on these postoperative pulmonary alterations are compared below. Respiratory alterations are less and recover more quickly following laparoscopy than after laparotomy. Vital capacity is reduced to 52% of the pre-operative value after a laparotomy, whereas it is reduced to only 75% of the pre-operative value after a laparoscopy.[26,27] Diaphragmatic function is altered less by laparoscopy than laparotomy as shown in recent report which failed to find any significant change in diaphragmatic function during quiet breathing after laparoscopic cholecystectomy.[28] Likewise FRC and residual volume (RV) remained normal during quiet breathing.[28] These data suggest that the risk of pulmonary complications might be decreased by laparoscopy compared to laparotomy. This is in agreement with studies suggesting that laparoscopic cholecystectomy is associated with a low rate (about 0.07%) of pulmonary complications.[29]

CARDIOVASCULAR CHANGES ASSOCIATED WITH LAPAROSCOPY

Effect of position

The increased hydrostatic pressure associated with the head-down position results in an increase venous return, central venous pressure and stroke index. Arterial blood pressure remains constant because concomitant baroreceptor reflex stimulation results in systemic vasodilation and bradycardia.[30,31] When the head-down tilt does not exceed 15°, the blood volume shift is too small to induce any clinically significant change in haemodynamics in healthy subjects.[32] Hence, haemodynamic changes induced by the Trendelenburg position are of little clinical significance.[33-35]

In patients with coronary disease or compromised ventricular function, increased central blood volume and central venous pressure are associated with deleterious effects such as increased myocardial oxygen consumption.[36] The head-down position increases intracranial and intraocular pressure. Therefore, the Trendelenburg position should be avoided in patients with increased intracranial pressure or acute glaucoma.

The head-up position results in blood pooling in the legs and decreased venous return. Consequently, cardiac output and blood pressure are decreased.[31,37] These decreases are proportional to the steepness of the tilt.[13]

Effect of increased intra-abdominal pressure

Earlier studies reported no significant haemodynamic alteration during laparoscopic procedures. These studies were performed during short gynaecological procedures in young healthy patients lying in the head-down position.[33,34] In contrast, all recent studies agree that laparoscopy is associated with a decreased cardiac output.[13,35,37-40] Differences in levels of intra-abdominal pressure, in the flow rate of insufflated gas, the timing of measurements, the anaesthetic technique and the patient position might account for these discrepancies. The decrease in cardiac output is proportional to the intra-abdominal pressure.[7,18] It can reach 50% of the pre-operative value.[37]

Cardiac output decrease is mainly related to a decreased stroke index since heart rate is not significantly affected by peritoneal insufflation. Decreased cardiac output can be related to decreased preload, increased afterload and alteration of myocardial function. So far myocardial function has not been studied during laparoscopy.

Decreased preload

Peritoneal insufflation of gas is associated with increased right atrial pressure. However, because part of the increased intra-abdominal pressure is transmitted to the thoracic cavity through the diaphragm, pressures obtained from a Swan Ganz or a central venous catheter no longer reflect venous return.[18,37,41,42] Transmural right atrial pressure, the actual indicator of venous return in these conditions, is in fact decreased. A decreased venous return is the result of a decreased blood flow in the inferior vena cava. This is because of blood pooling in the legs.[18,41-44]

Increased afterload

Shortly after peritoneal insufflation begins blood pressure increases while cardiac output decreases.[18,35,37,39] Hence, systemic vascular resistance (SVR) increases. SVR subsequently decreases but remains above the pre-operative value.[37] Compression of intra-abdominal vessels by increased intra-abdominal pressure may contribute to the increased SVR.[18,35,40] However, because it takes several minutes after exsufflation to return to pre-insufflation values, release of humoral factors has been suggested: catecholamines, renin, prostaglandins, vasopressin, etc.[35,39,45] Involvement of catecholamines is unlikely because their levels during laparoscopy are similar to those observed during laparotomy.[27] In addition, plasma noradrenaline concentration and renin activity are not altered by pneumo-peritoneum in patients breathing spontaneously.[42] A role for vasopressin is more likely since the time course of vasopressin levels and systemic vascular resistance are parallel.[46] Furthermore, vasopressin plasma levels correlate with changes in intra-abdominal pressure.

Regional blood flow

Increased intra-abdominal pressure decreases blood flow to the intra-abdominal organs, except the adrenal gland.[47–50] Splenic blood flow, in particular, is decreased and this decrease outlasts the pneumoperitoneum. Mesenteric and intestinal mucosal blood flow are also altered by increased intra-abdominal pressure.[47–49] The ensuing intestinal mucosal ischaemia results in a decreased intestinal mucosal pH and may delay the return of normal bowel function. Renal blood flow and glomerular filtration are decreased to 25% of the pre-operative value.[49] However, no adverse effect has been reported during laparoscopy in patients with impaired renal function. However, this is theoretically possible: renal failure has been described during increased intra-abdominal pressure from postoperative haemorrhage. Surgical decompression of the abdomen was associated with the resolution of acute renal failure.

Diaphragmatic blood flow is increased or unchanged by increases in intra-abdominal pressure.[48] Coronary blood flow is unchanged or increased in relation to cardiac output.[49,51] Intraperitoneal insufflation of CO_2 increases cerebral blood flow velocity and intracranial pressure, probably by an increased $Paco_2$.[52]

Haemodynamic changes seem well tolerated in healthy patients, as suggested by the normal venous O_2 saturation and lactate plasma levels observed during laparoscopic procedures in healthy patients.[37] Tolerance might be different in patients with impaired cardiac function, anaemia or hypovolaemia.

COMPLICATIONS OF LAPAROSCOPIC SURGICAL TECHNIQUES

As for any surgical technique, laparoscopy is not devoid of complications. Although morbidity and mortality are low, severe and sometimes lethal complications can occur. Most complications are related to the surgical technique and to the incompetence and/or inexperience of the surgeon. This has led some to state that laparoscopy is not dangerous but laparoscopists are.[53] The anaesthetist has to be aware of all potential complications in order to prevent and/or to treat them adequately.

The first morbidity-mortality studies about laparoscopy included patients undergoing gynaecological procedures. There is a large discrepancy between the published studies. In the early 1970s, the mortality rate was 2 in 10 000. Thereafter, it decreased significantly to reach 1 in 100 000 by the end of that decade.[54] Possible explanations for the improved outcome in patients undergoing surgical laparoscopic procedures include: better knowledge of the pathophysiologic changes associated with laparoscopy and training and better experience of the surgeons and anaesthetists. Although laparoscopy has only recently been introduced for abdominal procedures, the mortality rate after laparoscopy is similar to open laparotomy (0.2%).[55-57] The level of major complications is less than 2% after gastrointestinal laparoscopy in most studies.[53,55-57] Many of the major complications may necessitate conversion from laparoscopy to open laparotomy for adequate treatment.

Traumatic complications

Vascular trauma

Although unusual (±0.1% for gynaecological procedures;[53,58-62] 2% for abdominal surgery[63,64]), vascular injury is responsible for 30% of major complications of laparoscopic surgical procedures. Vessel injury can occur early during this procedure: i.e., as soon as the Veress needle is introduced. Injury to vessels in the abdominal wall can result in parietal haematoma and can lead to haemorrhagic shock. Major vessel (aorta, vena cava) trauma can be rapidly catastrophic and sometimes fatal. Vessels may also be injured in the retroperitoneal space. In such circumstances, the diagnosis is frequently delayed because a large volume of blood can be lost before intraperitoneal diffusion occurs.[58]

Abdominal viscera trauma

One-half of the complications necessitating a conversion from laparoscopy to an open laparotomy are abdominal viscera trauma.[61,62] They include hepatic and splenic tears and perforation of the stomach or the intestinal tract.[53,62] Gastric dilation secondary to ventilation by face mask might increase the risk of gastric perforation. Such injuries are often not recognized intraoperatively.[61,62,65] Untreated gastro-intestinal perforation can result in peritonitis, subdiaphragmatic abscess formation, septic shock and death.[29,63] Unrecognized splenic or hepatic trauma can induce haemorrhagic shock. Kidney, ureter and bladder trauma can also occur.[29,53,61,62]

Respiratory complications

Subcutaneous emphysema, pneumothorax, pneumomediastinum, pneumopericardium

Laparoscopy requires the creation of a pneumoperitoneum. This is obtained by gas (generally CO_2) insufflation in the peritoneal cavity and is associated with potential respiratory complications. Gas is insufflated in the peritoneal cavity via a Veress needle. If poorly inserted, this needle allows gas to pass into subcutaneous tissue and leads to the creation of subcutaneous emphysema.

Under pressure, the gas can move from the peritoneal cavity to the mediastinum, the pericardial or the pleural cavities, generating pneumomediastinum, pneumopericardium or pneumothorax which may or may not be associated with subcutaneous emphysema.[66-70] This movement of gas is possible through congenital foramina or defects in the diaphragm, especially at the great vessels or oesophageal hiatus. The increased alveolar pressure associated with the pneumoperitoneum may induce pre-existing emphysematous bullae to rupture, resulting in pneumothorax.[37] However, the most frequent cause of pneumothorax during laparoscopy is a pleural tear of surgical origin, e.g. during fundoplication for hiatus hernia.[71]

A pneumothorax should be suspected in patients with sudden or progressive hypoxaemia (cyanosis, decreased oxygen saturation), alteration of respiratory mechanics (increased peak airway pressure), and/or subcutaneous emphysema. The diagnosis is confirmed by auscultation or by observation of an abnormal diaphragmatic motion by the laparoscopist and is established with the demonstration of a visceral pleural line on the chest radiography. Although tube thoracostomy is the classical management for pneumothorax, one should consider the following before inserting chest tubes during a laparoscopy. Tube thoracostomy can compromise maintenance of the pneumoperitoneum and hence, the laparoscopic surgical procedure. In the absence of visceral pleural trauma, most intraoperative pneumothoraces occurring during a pneumoperitoneum will resolve spontaneously within 30 to 60 minutes after exsufflation, at least if the insufflated gas (such as CO_2) is rapidly diffusible.[68]

Hence, if a pneumothorax is diagnosed during a laparoscopy, one should increase FiO_2 to correct hypoxaemia, stop N_2O administration and decrease intra-abdominal pressure. The use of PEEP (5 cmH_2O) is associated with beneficial effects in the absence of pulmonary trauma.[71] A single needle drainage can be considered postoperatively if spontaneous resolution does not occur within one hour. Intra- or postoperative insertion of a thoracostomy tube should be avoided unless necessary.

Gas embolism

The most feared complication of gas insufflation in the peritoneal cavity is gas embolism[53,72] (ranging from 0 to 590 in 100 000 laparoscopies). It occurs more frequently when hysteroscopy is associated with laparoscopy.[73] Possible causes of gas embolism include: insufflation of gas into a vessel or an abdominal viscus due to a misplaced trocar or Veress needle, small bubbles of gas carried along in injured veins and large gas absorption into the portal circulation where bubbles can be formed and trapped.[72,74] These bubbles are released after peritoneal exsufflation and/or during mobilization. This latter mechanism would explain delayed occurrence of gas embolism.[75]

Symptoms and consequences of gas embolism are a function of the gas entry rate into the vessels, the size and the number of bubbles and the physical characteristics of the gas. Low rates of gas entry produce small bubbles that result in entrapment of gas in the pulmonary vessels. Higher rates of entry produce larger bubbles that form a 'gas lock' in the vena cava or in the right atrium.[76] The rate of gas insufflation during laparoscopy makes the latter more likely. Gas accumulation in the right heart and pulmonary vessels may result in high right atrial and ventricular pressure, decreased cardiac output, circulatory collapse and death. High right ventricular pressure can result in paradoxical embolism, even in the absence of patent foramen ovale, as a result of CO_2 in the cerebral and coronary circulation, with catastrophic consequences.[73,77–79]

Peritoneal insufflation has been performed with CO_2, N_2O and N_2. CO_2 is generally preferred because of its greater solubility in blood and rapid elimination by the lungs, in addition to its low cost, ready availability and non-flammability. The lethal dose of CO_2 in dogs is 25 ml/kg. This is equivalent to 1 l in human beings.[80] The inhalation of N_2O does not increase the size of CO_2 bubbles.[81]

During laparoscopy under general anaesthesia, gas embolism should be suspected in the presence of hypoxaemia, hypotension, tachycardia, ECG changes, jugular turgescence and circulatory collapse. Respiration can also be altered by gas embolism. Increased peak airway pressure, tachypnoea and desynchronization from the ventilator can be observed in patients with no muscle relaxation. Unlike air embolus, CO_2 embolus does not produce bronchoconstriction. In patients under general anaesthesia, immediate neurological symptoms are most often limited to bilateral mydriasis. At the end of anaesthesia, coma, delayed awakening, seizures, paresis or paralysis suggest CO_2 in the cerebral vessel: blindness results in 20% of cases.

A precordial or an oesophageal stethoscope may detect gas embolism early. Two or three seconds after the embolus of a limited volume of gas,[72] a metallic murmur can be heard. With increasing volume of gas, the classical 'millwheel murmur' occurs.[74,76]

The first haemodynamic change associated with gas embolism is an increase in pulmonary artery pressure (easily detected by a pulmonary artery or a Swan Ganz catheter).[82,83] The increase in pulmonary artery pressure is a function of the size of the embolus. Aspiration of gas or foaming blood by Swan Ganz catheter will confirm the diagnosis. However, the low incidence of clinically significant gas embolus during laparoscopies precludes the routine use of such an invasive monitoring.

Precordial Doppler probes can detect as little as 2 ml of gas passing through the right atrium.[82] Oesophageal Doppler is even more sensitive, detecting gas emboli as small as 0.5 ml.[84] Hence, Doppler probes allow the detection of gas embolism prior to physiological changes. However, the cost of this device and the low incidence of gas embolism preclude its routine use for laparoscopy.

Capnometry and/or capnography is one of the most valuable non-invasive techniques used to detect gas embolism, although the response time is longer than that of the auscultatory or Doppler methods.[85] $P_{ET}CO_2$ alterations during CO_2 embolism are biphasic. Small volumes of CO_2 embolus are excreted from the lung, increasing $P_{ET}CO_2$.[73,76] With increasing volumes of CO_2 embolus, $P_{ET}CO_2$ decreases owing to the decreased cardiac output and/or the enlargement of the physiological dead space that is secondary to the gas lock in the pulmonary artery.[86] Monitoring of the airway pressure is not helpful in detecting CO_2 embolism. Transcutaneous oximetry is not sensitive enough.

The incidence of gas embolism may be reduced by repeated and systematic aspiration tests to check that the Veress needle is correctly positioned. The use of CO_2, low rates of insufflation and low intra-abdominal pressure decrease the severity of the consequences of gas embolism. If the results of studies of gas embolism in neurosurgery can be extrapolated to intra-abdominal gas insufflation, fluid loading should decrease the incidence of gas embolism. The use of PEEP during coelioscopy is not recommended because it increases the incidence of paradoxical embolus and the risk of pulmonary barotrauma.

As soon as a gas embolus is suspected, insufflation gas must cease and the pneumoperitoneum released. The patient should be placed in Durants position (association of Trendelenburg and left lateral decubitus postion).[87] This posture helps prevent significant amounts of gas from entering the pulmonary vessels because the right ventricle outflow tract is uppermost.[76] Ventilator settings should be adjusted to increase CO_2 excretion. Increasing FiO_2 helps correct hypoxaemia. The cessation of N_2O administration increases CO_2 bubble resorption but does not reduce the size of these bubbles. If necessary, a central venous catheter may be inserted to aspirate gas and/or foamy blood.[74] The use of multiperforated catheters allows the aspiration of up to 70% of the gas: this is associated with an increased rate of survival and a shorter stay in the intensive care unit.

Haemodynamic conditions should be maintained by inotropic drugs and external cardiac massage should be initiated if necessary. A major effect of external cardiac massage is to reduce the size of the gas bubbles. If these measures are not effective, it is worth noting that internal cardiac massage and cardiopulmonary bypass have been successfully performed.[73]

Because ischaemia related to CO_2 embolism is brief, owing to the high solubility of CO_2 resulting in rapid absorption from the bloodstream, cerebral protective measures such as hypothermia or barbiturate administration may be beneficial.[88] Treatment with hyperbaric oxygen may be considered if neurological symptoms persist.

Endobronchial intubation

Intra-peritoneal insufflation of gas and the head-down position are associated with a cephalad shift of the diaphragm and intrathoracic organs. This shift may be associated with a movement of the tube in a mainstem bronchus.[37] The proximal tip of the tracheal tube should be firmly taped so the tube does not move in the trachea as the carina is displaced cephalad.[89] The tube should be carefully positioned so that it cuff is well above the carina and the position must be checked after creation of the pneumoperitoneum and after any change in patient position.

Aspiration of gastric contents

Theoretically, the increased intra-abdominal pressure associated with laparoscopy facilitates regurgitation. However, pressure at the lower oesophageal sphincter is increased more than gastric pressure.[90] The ensuing increased pressure gradient at the gastroesophageal junction should reduce the risk of regurgitation. However, the risk of regurgitation and acid aspiration persists because the volume and acidity of the gastric juice is sufficient to produce Mendelson's syndrome and because drugs and co-existing disease (e.g. hiatus hernia) may alter lower oesophageal sphincter tone. Therefore, pre-operative administration of antacids and H_2 receptors antagonists is recommended.[91,92]

Cardiovascular complications

Arrhythmia

Laparoscopy is known to be associated with a high incidence of cardiac irregularities.[93] Hypercapnia, hypoxia, haemodynamic changes and vagal reflexes are known to precipitate arrhythmias. In patients under halothane anaesthesia and breathing spontaneously, the incidence of arrhythmia is 27%.[93] If patients' lungs are mechanically ventilated and N_2O is used for insufflation – instead of CO_2 – thus resulting in a lower Pa_{CO_2}, the incidence of arrhythmia is 5%.[9] Because arrhythmias occur mainly in patients with a high CO_2, hypercapnia is considered as a major cause of arrhythmia during laparoscopy. Therefore, mechanical ventilation and use of enflurane or isoflurane, which are less arrhythmogenic than halothane, are recommended.[94,95]

Hypoxia is seldom observed in patients undergoing laparoscopy. It can be the consequence of either hypoventilation, in spontaneously breathing patients, or ventilation-perfusion mismatch. The latter is favoured by high intra-abdominal pressures. Mechanical ventilation, increased FiO_2, optimization of ventilatory settings and reduction of intra-abdominal pressure helps to correct hypoxaemia.

Peritoneal traction, abdominal organ displacement and electrocoagulation of fallopian tubes increase vagal tone and result in cardiac arrhythmias, bradycardia or circulatory collapse.[96-98] If a vagal reaction occurs, one should consider stopping insufflation and administering atropine. Anaesthesia may be deepened as soon as normal haemodynamic conditions are restored. Haemodynamic changes which occur during intraperitoneal insufflation of gas is another cause of irregularity, especially in patients with concomitant cardiovascular disease. Last but not least, arrhythmia may also be the first sign of a gas embolus.

Per-operative collapse

The decreased venous return associated with intraperitoneal insufflation of gas can result in circulatory collapse. Co-existing cardiovascular disease, pre-operative hypovolaemia, intra-operative haemorrhage and excessive intra-abdominal pressure all favour the likelihood of circulatory arrest.

Nerve injury

Changes in patient position can result in nerve compression or overextension.[53] Special attention must be paid to prevention of brachial plexus compression by shoulder braces in the head-down position (shoulder braces should face the coracoid process and only moderate tilt should be used). Similarly, inadequate fixation of the lower limbs can result in neuropathies and/or compartment syndrome.[99-101]

ANAESTHETIC MANAGEMENT

Patient selection

There are no prospective studies comparing peri-operative mortality and morbidity between laparoscopic procedures and open surgery in order to draw conclusions over patient selection.

Increases in intra-abdominal pressure preclude laparoscopic procedures in patients with intraperitoneal shunt or peritoneo-jugular shunts. Likewise, laparoscopy is contraindicated in patients with acute glaucoma and in patients with raised intracranial pressure because intraperitoneal insufflation of gas is associated with increased intraocular pressure, increased cerebral blood flow velocity and increased intracranial pressure. In contrast, laparoscopy is no more dangerous than laparotomy in obese patients.[25]

In patients with severe respiratory disease, laparoscopy is associated with a higher risk of pneumothorax and inadequate gas exchange during the pneumoperitoneum. However, this may be offset by the reduced post-operative respiratory dysfunction and the potential decrease of pulmonary complications.[29]

Haemodynamic changes associated with the pneumoperitoneum (increased afterload, decreased venous return and cardiac output) might be deleterious in patients with compromized ventricular function and in patients with ischaemic cardiac disease. Hence, the anaesthetist has to weigh up the risk of intraoperative cardiac complications and the postoperative benefits of laparoscopy.

Use of an intra-abdominal suspension umbrella instead of abdominal insufflation of gas for laparoscopy may result in fewer side-effects and could be an alternative in patients with concomitant diseases. If insufflation of gas is used, the insufflation and exsufflation should be as slow and as smooth as possible.[102] Intra-abdominal pressure must be carefully monitored and maintained as low as possible.

Pre-operative medication

The choice of pre-operative medication should be adapted to type and length of surgery as well as the patients' needs. Atropine must be administered intravenously before induction of anaesthesia to prevent vagal reactions associated with laparoscopic surgery. Antacids and H_2–receptor antagonists are recommended by some to reduce the risk of regurgitation and acid aspiration.[91,92] Deep vein thrombosis prevention (antistasis stockings and low molecular weight heparin) is mandatary because the pneumoperitoneum is associated with decreased blood flow in the lower limbs.[103] Pre-operative administration of clonidine or other α_2 agonists reduce the haemodynamic and stress response to surgery.[104] Peri-operative administration of antiemetic drugs help reduce postoperative nausea.[105,106] Non-steroidal anti-inflammatory drugs administered peri-operatively help reduce postoperative pain. The ensuing reduction of postoperative consumption of opioids will also contribute to the reduction of postoperative nausea and vomiting.

Monitoring

Routine intra-operative monitoring of patients undergoing laparoscopy includes non-invasive arterial blood pressure measurement, continuous ECG, capnometry and pulse oximetry. During laparoscopy, hypoxaemia can result from excessive intra-abdominal pressure, pneumothorax, endobronchial intubation, gas embolus and haemoglobinopathy.

End-tidal $P_{ET}CO_2$ varies with cardiac output, minute ventilation and $\dot{V}CO_2$. Hence, $P_{ET}CO_2$ changes may be difficult to interpret. CO_2 embolus is associated with a biphasic change in $P_{ET}CO_2$: the initial increase results from the increased CO_2 elimination followed by a decrease related to the decreased cardiac output. A progressive increase in $P_{ET}CO_2$ reveals endobronchial intubation, subcutaneous emphysema or pneumothorax. It is worth pointing out that $(a-A)D_{CO_2}$ varies during laparoscopy and differs from one patient to another. Because changes in $(a-A)D_{CO_2}$ are greater in patients with cardiac and/or respiratory disease, radial artery cannulation should be considered for arterial blood gas analysis in these patients. Cardiac filling pressures monitoring by a Swan Ganz catheter might be useful in patients with heart disease. However, changes in intrathoracic pressures associated with pneumoperitoneum render the interpretation of the wedge and right atrial pressures difficult. Transoesophageal echocardiography are more valuable in such patients. Thoracic compliance and/or airway pressure monitoring are also essential. During intra-peritoneal gas insufflation, the cephalad shift of the diaphragm and decreased thoracopulmonary compliance result in increased airway pressure. Pneumothorax, subcutaneous emphysema and endobronchial intubation are associated with large increases in airway pressure. ST segment monitoring of the ECG is probably of little value during laparoscopy because cephalad shift of the diaphragm modifies the heart axis. An oesophageal stethoscope and/or a precordial ultrasound Doppler have been advocated by some.

For long surgical procedures, body temperature and muscle relaxation monitoring are helpful. Haemodynamic and respiratory monitoring should be continued in the recovery room since cardiovascular and ventilatory changes outlast the laparoscopic surgical procedure.

Aanaesthetic technique

Laparoscopy has been performed successfully and safely under local, regional and general anaesthesia.

Local anaesthesia decreases the side effects of general anaesthesia such as muscle pain, sore throat, postoperative nausea, vomiting etc.,[107] and allows verbal contact with the patient. However, this anaesthetic technique is frequently associated with patient anxiety, pain, etc. Hence, it requires supplementary intravenous sedation which can result in severe hypoxaemia and hypercapnia.[108] An experienced surgical team, a skilled surgeon and a co-operative patient are thus essential for the success of this technique. In addition, local anaesthesia should not be used for laparoscopic procedures necessitating extensive organ manipulation, numerous puncture sites or high intra-abdominal pressure. Indeed, these procedures would be associated with pain and breathing difficulties.

Regional anaesthesia has been proposed for gynaecological laparoscopy. It has the same advantages as local anaesthesia, such as avoidance of muscle pain and sore throat. In patients under epidural anaesthesia, ventilatory variables are unaffected by body position.[15] Intraperitoneal insufflation of CO_2 results in increased minute ventilation and respiratory rate so that $Paco_2$ remains constant.[15] The cardiovascular changes associated with epidural anaesthesia for laparoscopy have so far not been assessed. However, one can speculate that sympathetic blockade associated with epidural anaesthesia can offset the increase in afterload associated with the pneumoperitoneum. On the other hand, the sympathetic blockade may exaggerate the decrease in venous return and promote the occurrence of vagal reflexes. Epidural blockade does not provide complete analgesia during laparoscopy: shoulder pain secondary to diaphragmatic irritation by insufflated gas is mediated by the phrenic nerve.[109] Therefore, use of epidural anaesthesia for laparoscopy should be restricted to short procedures performed by skilled surgeons, in co-operative patients. For instance, regional anaesthesia has never been advocated for laparoscopic cholecystectomy, except for patients with cystic fibrosis.[110]

General anaesthesia, endotracheal intubation and mechanical ventilation is the technique of choice for laparoscopic surgical procedures. This method prevents hypoventilation and the use of a tracheal tube helps reduce the likelihood of aspiration of gastric contents. In addition, it provides optimal operative conditions and complete analgesia. Thiopentone remains the agent most frequently used to induce anaesthesia for laparoscopy. Ketamine, diazepam, etomidate and propofol have been advocated for induction and maintenance of anaesthesia (total intravenous anaesthesia). Propofol is associated with quick recovery and with less postoperative nausea and vomiting (PONV).[111] Anaesthesia can also be maintained with inhalational anaesthetics. The use of N_2O during laparoscopic surgery remains controversial because it is thought to increase PONV and to produce bowel distension. However, there is no conclusive evidence so far that N_2O alters surgical conditions during laparoscopic procedures or increases the incidence of PONV. Therefore, N_2O should still be considered as a useful adjuvant for maintenance of general anaesthesia during laparoscopic procedures. In the instance of bowel perforation, nitrous oxide can reach concentrations in the peritoneal cavity that can support combustion of bowel gas.[112] Hence, if a bowel perforation is recognized, N_2O should be removed from the anaesthetic mixture and the peritoneal cavity purged with CO_2.

Cardiac function is less altered by isoflurane than by enflurane or halothane. In the presence of hypercapnia, arrythmias occur less often when isoflurane is administered than when halothane is used. Moreover, the vasodilating properties of isoflurane reduces the increase in the systemic vascular resistance observed during the pneumoperitoneum. Hence, isoflurane is the volatile anaesthetic agent of choice for laparoscopic procedures: sevoflurane and desflurane are being assessed.

During pneumoperitoneum, minute ventilation must be increased by 15 to 50% to maintain $P_{ET}co_2$ between 4.0–4.7 kPa (30 and 35 mmHg). However, larger minute ventilation increases may result in subcutaneous emphysema; in order to minimize barotrauma, the increase in minute ventilation should be obtained by increasing respiratory rate rather than by increasing tidal volume.

For short laparoscopic procedures by experienced surgeons using low intra-abdominal pressures and moderate tilt in healthy patients, tracheal intubation and mechanical ventilation may not be essential. However, it should be kept in mind that more than 50% of anaesthetic deaths are related to hypoventilation. Hence, in spontaneously breathing patients undergoing laparoscopy, continuous monitoring of $P_{ET}CO_2$ and SpO_2 is crucial.

The use of laryngeal mask airway during laparoscopy is still controversial.[113,114] Laryngeal masks do not prevent pulmonary aspiration of gastric content. Moreover, intra-peritoneal insufflation of gas results in decreased thoracopulmonary compliance and peak airway pressure above 20 mmHg during mechanical ventilation. Because air leaks usually occur when a laryngeal mask is used at this pressure, the laryngeal mask should be used only in very carefully selected patients.[106,114,115]

Postoperative period

Postoperative O_2 administration is mandatory after laparoscopic procedures.[116] Indeed, postoperative increase in O_2 consumption and respiratory dysfunction can result in hypoxaemia. Special attention needs to be paid to prevent and/or treat PONV and pain.[27]

KEY POINTS

- Advantages of laparoscopy are multiple and explain its ever-increasing popularity. They include: less trauma, less pain, less postoperative ileus, less postoperative pulmonary dysfunction, quicker recovery and a shorter hospital stay.
- Laparoscopy is not devoid of side-effects and complications can lead to death.
- Complications may be related to pathophysiological changes associated with intraperitoneal gas insufflation and with patient positioning. Other complications are due to the surgical technique.
- Pathophysiological cardiorespiratory changes associated with laparoscopy have been studied in healthy patients. Whether these results are extensible to patients with co-existing disease remains to be determined.
- Laparoscopy is well-tolerated by the young and healthy. Tolerance of older and sicker patients who present for laparoscopy is still unknown.
- General anaesthesia with intubation and mechanical ventilation is the technique of choice for laparoscopic procedures. Use of the laryngeal mask airway might be safe in selected patients. Spontaneous breathing should be restricted to very short laparoscopic procedures. Likewise, epidural anaesthesia should be limited to quick lower abdominal or gynaecological procedures.

- Intravenous sedation during laparoscopy can result in profound alterations in gas exchange.

REFERENCES

1. Bernheim B M. Organoscopy: cystoscopy of the abdominal cavity. Ann Surg 1911; 53: 764
2. Steptoe P C. Laparoscopy in gynaecology. ES Livingstone, London, 1967: p 104
3. Perissat J, Collet D R, Belliart R. Gallstone: Laparoscopic treatment, intracorporeal lithotripsy followed by cholecystostomy or cholecystectomy – a personal technique. Endoscopy 1989; 21: 373–374
4. Reddick E J, Olsen D O. Laparoscopic laser cholecystectomy. A comparison with mini-lap cholecystecomy. Surg Endosc 1989; 3: 131–133
5. Way L W. Changing therapy for gallstone disease. N Engl J Med 1990; 323: 1273–1274
6. Neugebauer E, Troidl H, Spangenberger W et al. The cholecystectomy Study Group: Conventional versus laparoscopic cholecystectomy and the randomized controlled trial. Br J Surg 1991; 78: 150–154
7. Dubois F, Berthelot G, Levard H. Laparoscopic cholecystectomy: Historical perspective and personal experience. Surg Laparoscop Endosc 1991; 1: 52–57
8. Alexander G D, Noe F E, Brown E M. Anesthesia for pelvic laparoscopy. Anesth Analg 1969; 48: 14–18
9. Scott D B, Julian D G. Observations on cardiac arrythmias during laparoscopy. Br Med J 1972; 1: 411–414
10. Baratz R A, Karis J H. Blood gas studies during laparoscopy under general anaesthesia. Anesthesiology 1969; 30: 463–464
11. Cunningham A J, Schlanger M. Intraoperative hypoxemia complicating laparoscopic cholecystectomy in a patient with sickle hemoglobinopathy. Anesth Analg 1992; 75: 838–843
12. Schmid E R, Rehder K. General anesthesia and the chest wall. Anesthesiology 1981; 55: 668–675
13. Nyarwaya J B, Samii K, Mazoit J X, de Watteville J C. Are pulse oximetric and capnographic monitoring reliable during laparoscopic surgery for cholecystectomy? Anesthesiology 1991; 75: A453
14. Brown D R, Fishburne J I, Roberson V O, Hulka J F. Ventilatory and blood gas changes during laparoscopy with local anaesthesia. Am J Obstet Gynecol 1976; 24: 741–745
15. Ciofolo M J, Clergue F, Seebacher J et al. Ventilatory effects of laparoscopy under epidural anesthesia. Anesth Analg 1990; 70: 357–361
16. Nunn J F. Carbon dioxide. In: Nunn J F (ed) Applied Respiratory Physiology, 3rd edn. Butterworth, London, 1987: 207–237
17. Lister D R, Rudston-Brown B, Warriner B et al. Carbon dioxide absorption is not linearly related to intraperitoneal carbon dioxide insufflation pressure in pigs. Anesthesiology 1994; 80: 129–136
18. Ivankovich A D, Miletich D J, Albrecht R F et al. Cardiovascular effects of intraperitoneal insufflation with carbon dioxide and nitrous oxide in the dog. Anesthesiology 1975; 42: 281–287
19. Magno R, Medegard A, Bengtsson R, Tronstad S E. Acid-base balance during laparoscopy. Acta Obstet Gynecol Scand 1979; 58: 81–85
20. Hodgson C, McClelland M A, Newton J R. Some effects of the peritoneal insufflation of carbon dioxide at laparoscopy. Anesthesia 1970; 25: 382–390
21. Joris J, Ledoux D, Honor'e P, Lamy M. Ventilatory effects of CO_2 insufflation during laparoscopic cholecystectomy. Anesthesiology 1991; 75 (Suppl): A121
22. Puri G D, Singh H. Ventilatory effects of laparoscopy under general anesthesia. Br J Anaesth 1992; 68: 211
23. Sha M, Ohmura A, Yamada M. Diaphragm function and pulmonary complications after laparoscopic cholecystectomy. Anesthesiology 1991; 75 (suppl.): A255

24. Wittgen C W, Andrus C H, Fitzgerald S D et al. Analysis of the hemodynamic and ventilatory effect of laparoscopic cholecystectomy. Arch Surg 1991; 126: 997–1000
25. Bromberg N, Matusak J P, Mahieu G et al. Comparasion des mesures t'el'e-expiratoires, transcutane'es et arte'rielles du CO_2 au cours de la chole'cystectomie par laparoscopie. Ann Fr Anaesth Re'anim 1992; 32 (suppl): R2
26. Frazee R C, Roberts J W, Okeson G C et al. Open versus laparoscopic cholecystectomy. A comparison of postoperative pulmonary function. Ann Surg 1991; 213: 651–653
27. Joris J, Cigarini I, Legrand M et al. Metabolic and respiratory changes after cholecystectomy performed via laparotomy or laparoscopy. Br J Anaesth 1992; 69: 341–345
28. Couture J G, Chartrand D, Gagner M, Bellemare F. Diaphragmatic and abdominal muscle activity after endoscopic cholecystectomy. Anesth Analg 1994; 78: 733–739
29. The Southem Surgeons Club. A prospective analysis of 1,518 laparoscopic cholecys-tectomie. N Engl J Med 1991; 324: 1073–1078
30. Sibbald W J, Paterson N A M, Holliday R L, Baskerville J. The Trendelenburg position: hemodynamic effects in hypotensive and normotensive patients. Crit Care Med 1979; 7: 218–224
31. Yukinobu A, Nishikawa T. Heart rate responses to body tilt during spinal anesthesia. Anesth Analg 1991; 73: 385–390
32. Bivins H G, Knopp R, dos Santos P A L. Blood volume distribution in the Trendelenburg position. Ann Emerg Med 1985; 14: 641–643
33. Motew M, Ivankovich A, Bieniarz J et al. Cardiovascular effects and acid-base and blood gas changes during laparoscopy. Am J Obstet Gynecol 1973; 115: 1002–1012
34. Lenz R J, Thomas T A, Wilkins D G. Cardiovascular changes during laparoscopy: studies of stroke volume and cardiac output using impedance cardiography. Anaesthesia 1976; 31: 4–12
35. Torrielli R, Cesarini M, Winnock S et al. Modifications hémodynamiques durant la coelioscopie: étude menie par bio-impédance électrique thoracique. Can J Anaesth 1990; 37: 46–51
36. Wilcox S, Vandam L D. Alas, poor Trendelenburg and his position! A critique of its use and effectiveness. Anesth Analg 1988, 67: 574–578
37. Joris J L, Noirot D P, Legrand M J et al. Hemodynamic changes during laparoscopic cholecystectomy. Anesth Analg 1993; 76: 1067–1071
38. MacKenzie R, Wadhwa R K, Bedger R C. Non invasive measurement of cardiac output during laparoscopy. J Reprod Med 1980; 24: 247–250
39. Schoeffler P, Haberer J P, Manhes H et al. Répercussions circulatoires et ventilatoires de la coelioscopie chez l'obe'se. Ann Fr Anaesth Re'anim 1984; 3: 10–15
40. Johannsen G, Andersen M, Juhl B. The effect of general anaesthesia on the haemodynamic events during laparoscopy with CO_2 insufflation. Acta Anaesthesiol Scand 1989; 33: 132–136
41. Diamant M, Benumof J, Saidman L J. Hemodynamics of increased intra-abdominal pressure: interaction with hypovolemia and halothane anesthesia. Anesthesiology 1978; 48: 23–27
42. Solis-Herruzo J A, Moreno D, Gonzalez A et al. Effect of intrathoracic pressure on plasma arginine vasopressin levels. Gastroenterology 1991; 101: 607–617
43. Rubinson R M, Vasko J S, Doppman J L, McRow A G. Inferior vena cava obstruction from increased intra-abdominal pressure. Arch Surg 1967; 94: 766–770
44. Richardson D J, Trinkli J K. Haemodynamic and respiratory alterations with increased intra-abdominal pressure. J Surg Res 1976; 20: 401–404
45. Marshall R L, Jebson P J R, Davie I T, Scott D B. Circulatory effects of peritoneal insufflation with nitrous oxide. Br J Anaesth 1972; 44: 1183–1187
46. Joris J, Lamy M. Neuroendocrine changes during pneumoperitoneum for laparoscopic cholecystectomy. Br J Anaesth 1993; 70 (suppl): A33
47. Ring J C, Smith-Wright D L, Einzing S et al. Effects of acute tense abdominal distension on regional blood flow and renal functions. Crit Care Med 1981; 12: 222
48. Masey S A, Koehler R C, Buck J R et al. Effect of abdominal distension on central and regional hemodynamics in neonatal lambs. Ped Res 1985; 19: 1244–1249

49. Caldwell C B, Ricotta J J. Changes in visceral blood flow with elevated intra-abdominal pressure. J Surg Res 1987; 43: 14–20
50. Diebel L N, Dulchavsky S A, Wilson R F. Effect of increased intra-abdominal pressure on mesenteric arterial and intestinal mucosal blood flow. J Trauma 1992; 33: 45–49
51. Lehot J J, Leone B J, Foëx P. Effects of altered PaO_2 and $Paco_2$ on left ventricular function and coronary hemodynamics in sheep. Anesth Analg 1991; 72: 737–743
52. Fujii Y, Tanaka H, Tsuruokat S et al. Middle cerebral arterial blood flow velocity increases during laparoscopic cholecystectomy. Anesth Analg 1994; 78: 80–83
53. Mintz M. Le risque et la prophylaxie des accidents en coelioscopie gynécologique: enquête portant sur 100 000 cas. J Gynecol Obstet Biol Reprod 1976; 5: 681
54. Semm K. Statistical survey of gynecological laparoscopy pelviscopy in Germany. Endoscopy 1979; 11: 101–106
55. Cuschieri A, Dubois F, Mouriel J et al. The European experience with laparoscopic cholecystectomy. Am J Surg 1991; 161: 385–387
56. Litwin D E M, Girotti M J, Poulin E C et al. Laparoscopic cholecystectomy: trans-Canada experience with 2201 cases. Can J Surg 1992; 35: 291–296
57. Strasberg S M, Sanabria J R, Clavien P A. Complications of laparoscopic cholecystectomy. Can J Surg 1992; 35: 275–280
58. Peterson H B, Hulka J F, Phillips J M. American Association of Gynecologic Laparoscopists' 1988 Membership Survey on operative laparoscopy. J Reprod Med 1990; 35: 587–589
59. Phillips J M, Hulka J F, Peterson H B. American Association of Gynecologic Laparoscopists' Membership Survey. J Reprod Med 1984; 29: 592–594
60. Von Theobald P, Marie G, Herlicoviez M, Levy G. Morbidité et mortalité de la coelioscopie. Etude rétrospective d'une série de 1429 cas. Rev Fr Gynécol Obstet 1989; 85: 611–614
61. Chapron C, Querleu D, Mage G et al. Complications de la coeliochirurgie gynécologique. J Gynécol Obstet Biol Reprod 1992; 21: 207–213
62. Querleu D, Chevalier L, Chapron C, Bruhat M A. Complications de la coeliochirurgie gynécologique. J Obstet Gynecol 1993; 7: 57–65
63. Collet D, Crozat T, Alhi S. Complications de la cholécystectomie coelioscopique. L'enquête de la SFCERO. Lyon Chir 1991, 87: 463–466
64. Francois Y, Braillon G, Cuilleret J. Morbidité de la cholécystectomie percoelioscopique. Etude de la Société de Chirurgie de Lyon: 1 060 observations. Lyon Chir 1991, 87: 456–463
65. Peterson H B, Destefano F, Rubin G L, et al. Deaths attributable to tubal sterilization in the United States. Am J Obstet Gynecol 1983, 146: 131–136
66. Whiston R J, Eggers K A, Movus R W, Stamatakis J D. Tension pneumothorax during laparoscopic cholecystectomy. Br J Surg 1991; 78: 1325
67. Doctor N H, Hussain Z. Bilateral pneumothorax associated with laparoscopy: a case report of a rare hazard and review of literature. Anaesthesia 1973; 28: 75–81
68. Batra M S, Discoll J J, Coburn W A, Marks W M. Evanescent nitrous oxide pneumothorax after laparoscopy. Anaesth Analg 1983; 62: 1121–1123
69. Spielman F J. Laparoscopic survey. In: Hood D D, Kirby R R, Brown D L (eds) Problems in anesthesia: anesthesia in obstetrics and gynecology. Lippincott, Philadelphia 1989; vol. 3
70. Knos G B, Sung Y F, Toledo A. Pneumopericardium associated with laparoscopy. J Clin Anaesth 1991; 3: 56–59
71. Chiche J D, Joris J, Lamy M. Peep for treatment of intraoperative pneumothorax during laparoscopic fundoplication. Br J Anaesth 1994; 72 (suppl. 1): A38
72. Hynes S R, Marshall R L. Venous gas embolism during gynaecologycal laparoscopy. Can J Anaesth 1992; 39: 748–749
73. Diakun T A. Carbon dioxide embolism: successful resuscitation with cardio-pulmonary bypass. Anesthesiology 1991; 74: 1151–1153
74. Yacoub O F, Cardona I, Coveler L A, Dodson M G. Carbon dioxide embolism during laparoscopy. Anesthesiology 1982; 57: 533–535
75. Root B, Levy M N, Pollack S et al. Gas embolism death after laparoscopy delayed by trapping in the portal circulation. Anesth Analg 1978; 57: 232–237

76. Shulman D, Aronson H B. Capnography in the early diagnosis of carbon dioxide embolism during laparoscopy. Can J Anaesth 1984; 31: 455–459
77. Butler B D, Hills B A. Transpulmonary passage of venous air emboli. J Appl Physiol 1985; 59: 543–547
78. McGrath B J, Zimmerman J E, Williams J F, Parmet J. Carbon dioxide embolism treated with hyperbaric oxygen. Can J Anaesth 1989; 36: 586–589
79. Albin M S, Ritter R R, Pruett C E, Kalff K. Venous air embolism during lumbar laminectomy in the prone position: report of three cases. Anesth Analg 1991; 73: 346–349
80. Graff T D, Arbegast N R, Philipps O C et al. Gas embolism: a comparative study of air and carbon dioxide as embolic agents in the systemic venous system. Am J Obstet Gynecol 1959; 78: 259
81. Losasso T J, Muzzi D A, Dietz N M, Cucchiara R F. Fifty percent nitrous oxide does not increase the risk of venous air embolism in the neurological patients operated upon in the sitting position. Anesthesiology 1992; 77: 21–30
82. English J B, Westenskow D, Hodges M R, Stanley T H. Comparison of venous air embolism monitoring methods in supine dogs. Anesthesiology 1978; 48: 425–429
83. Marshall W K, Bedford R F. Use of pulmonary artery catheter for detection and treatment of venous air embolism. Anesthesiology 1980; 52: 131–134
84. Martin R J, Colley P S. Evaluation of transoesophageal Doppler detection of air embolism in dogs. Anesthesiology 1983, 58: 117–123
85. Ostman P L, Pantle-Fisher F H, Faure E A, Glosten B. Circulatory collapse during laparoscopy. J Clin Anaesth 1990; 2: 129–132
86. Oppenheimer M J, Durant T M, Stauffer H M et al. In vivo visualization of intracardiac structures with gaseous carbon dioxide. Am J Physiol 1956; 186: 325–334
87. Alvaran S B, Toung J K, Graff T E, Benson D W. Venous air embolism: comparative merits of external cardiac massage intracardiac aspiration, and left lateral decubitus position. Anesth Analg 1978; 57: 166–170
88. Dietrich E B, Koopot R, Male A, Diess N. Successful reverse of brain damage from iatrogenic air embolism. Surg Gynecol Obstet 1982; 154: 572–575
89. Heinonen J, Takki S, Tammisto T. Effect of the Trendelenburg tilt and other procedures on the position of endotracheal tubes. Lancet 1969; i: 850–853
90. Jones M J, Mitchell R W, Hindocha N. Effect of increased intra-abdominal pressure during laparoscopy on the lower esophageal sphincter. Anesth Analg 1989; 68: 63–65
91. Duffy B L. Regurgitation during pelvic laparoscopy. Br J Anaesth 1979; 51: 1089–1090
92. Tay H S, Chiu H H. Acid aspiration during laparoscopy. Anaesth Intensive Care 1989, 6: 314
93. Scott D B. Some effects of peritoneal insufflation of carbon dioxide at laparoscopy. Anaesthesia 1970; 25: 590–593
94. Desmond J, Gordon R A. Ventilation in patients anaesthetized for laparoscopy. Can J Anaesth 1970; 17: 378–387
95. Harris M N E, Plantevin O M, Crowther A. Cardiac arrhythmias during anaesthesia for laparoscopy. Br J Anaesth 1984; 56: 1213–1217
96. Carmichael D E. Laparoscopy – cardiac considerations. Fertil Steril 1971; 22: 69–70
97. Brantley J C, Riley P M. Cardiovascular collapse during laparoscopy: a report of two cases. Am J Obstet Gynecol 1988; 159: 735–737
98. Myles P. Arrythmias during laparoscopy. Br J Anaesth 1989; 63: 365
99. Lydon J C, Spielman F J. Bilateral compartment syndrome following prolonged surgery in the lithotomy position. Anesthesiology 1984; 60: 236–238
100. Montgomery C J, Ready L B. Epidural opioid analgesia does not obscure diagnosis of compartment syndrome resulting from prolonged lithotomy position. Anesthesiology 1991; 75: 541–543
101. Johnston R V, Lawson N W, Nealon W H. Lower extremity neuropathy after laparoscopic cholecystectomy. Anesthesiology 1992; 77: 835
102. Baraka A. Cardiovascular collapse after carbon dioxide exsufflation in a patient undergoing laparoscopic cholecystectomy. Anesth Analg 1994; 78: 603

103. Beebe D S, McNevin M P, Belani K G et al. Evidence of venous stasis after abdominal insufflation for laparoscopic cholecystectomy. Anesthesiology 1992; 77 (suppl.): A148

104. Aho M, Lehtinen A M, Laatikainen T, Lortila K. Effects of intramuscular clonidine on hemodynamic and plasma β-endorphin responses to gynecologic laparoscopy. Anesthesiology 1990; 72: 797–802

105. Raphael J H, Norton A C. Antiemetic efficacy of prophylactic ondansetron in laparoscopic surgery: randomized, double-blind comparison with metoclopramide. Br J Anaesth 1993; 71: 845–848

106. Malins A F, Cooper G M. Laparoscopy and the laryngeal mask airway. Br J Anaesth 1994; 73: 121

107. Peterson H B, Hulka J, Spielman F J et al. Local versus general anesthesia for laparoscopic sterilization. A randomized study. Obstet Gynecol 1987; 70: 903–908

108. Brady C E, Harkleroad L E, Pierson W P. Alteration in oxygen saturation and ventilation after intravenous sedation for peritoneoscopy. Arch Intern Med 1989; 149: 1029

109. Lefebvre G, Vauthier-Brouzes D, Darbois Y et al. La coelioscopie sous anaesthésie péridurale: technique, indications, résultats à propos de 220 cas. J Gynecol Obstet Biol Reprod 1991; 20: 355–360

110. Edelman D S. Laparoscopic cholecystectomy under continuous epidural anesthésia in patients with cystic fibrosis (letter). Am J Dis Child 1991; 145: 723–724

111. Borgeat A, Wilder-Smith O H G, Saiah M, Rifat K. Subhypnotic doses of propofol possess direct antiemetic properties. Anesth Analg 1992; 74: 359–341

112. Neuman G G, Sidebotham G, Negoianu E et al. Laparoscopy explosion hazards with nitrous oxide. Anesthesiology 1993; 78: 875–879

113. Wilkinson P A, Cyna A M, MacLeod D M et al. The laryngeal mask: cautionary tales. Anesthesia 1990; 45: 167–168

114. Brimacombe J, Shorney N. Laparoscopy and the laryngeal mask airway? Anaesth Int Care 1992; 20: 245–246

115. Swann D G, Spens H, Edwards S A, Chesnut R J. Anaesthesia for gynaecological laparoscopy – a comparison between the laryngeal mask airway and tracheal intubation. Anaesthesia 1993; 48: 431–434

116. Vegfor M, Cederholm I, Lennmarken C, Lvftrvm A. Should oxygen be administered after laparoscopy in healthy patients? Acta Anaesthesiol Scand 1988; 32: 350

4

Anaesthesia and analgesia for caesarean section

G. Lyons

Caesarean section is a common operation; included by Guardian Health insurance company in its top 100 procedures, some 93 000 are performed every year in the United Kingdom.[1] In the United States in 1985, of 20 million anaesthetics, 4.4% (877 000) were given for caesarean section.[2] The rate of caesarean delivery has increased in all the countries of the Western world. In the United Kingdom in 1992, the rate was over 13%, but with considerable regional variation. In the United States in 1988, the rate was 24.7%, and in many European countries rates vary between 10% and 20%. Reasons for the increasing rate in the United Kingdom may be because the operation is becoming safer, on the one hand, while labour becomes more litigation prone on the other.[3] Negligence is more likely to be alleged when a caesarean section is delayed or not performed. For every 40 of such claims notified to the Medical Defence Union, there was only one alleging that the operation was unnecessary.[4] Nevertheless, a feeling exists that perhaps current trends are undesirable. The Netherlands seem able to cope with a caesarean delivery rate of less than 10%,[3] but it is possible that current rates could be in the interests of mother and baby.[5]

MORTALITY AND MORBIDITY

In 1994 the Report on Confidential Enquiries into Maternal Deaths in the United Kingdom for the years 1988–90 was published. This confirmed that anaesthesia has declined in importance from 13% to 3% of all maternal deaths. Of the five deaths reported, three occurred in association with caesarean section, implicating aspiration of gastric contents, poor airway control, and poor postoperative care.[1] Recommendations made for improving care are listed below.

- The provision of CO_2 analysers in all locations where general anaesthetics are given.
- Administration of H_2 receptor antagonists to patients who may require anaesthesia, and those with pre-eclampsia.
- Administration of nonparticulate antacids before induction of general anaesthesia.

- Emptying of the stomach before tracheal extubation via a gastric tube to minimize the risks of postoperative aspiration.
- Early insertion of large gauge intravenous cannulae and monitoring of central venous pressure (CVP) when severe blood loss is observed or suspected.
- Improvements in standards of postoperative care.
- Greater reliance upon departmental guidelines including calling for senior assistance.
- Use of pulse oximetry perioperatively to detect pulmonary complications.

In a prominent editorial, a number of questions raised by these recommendations were asked.[6] Should antacid prophylaxis be extended to all in labour, should a nasogastric tube be considered standard practice during general anaesthesia and should CVP be measured continuously rather than intermittently? If the last question asks if electronic measurement is superior to manometric, then virtually every intensive care unit in the United Kingdom is likely to give a positive answer. The notion that the stomach should be emptied intraoperatively by a gastric tube will be new to some units. Use of a nasogastric tube implies pre-operative use on an awake patient, a practice that has proved unpopular with patients and anaesthetists. In drawing attention to the potential for postoperative aspiration, and advocating the intraoperative use of a gastric tube, we are given both the problem and the solution. With an anaesthetised patient the objections disappear. Given that the removal of particulate gastric contents will be governed by the internal diameter of the tube, a large bore orogastric tube is required. At the same time gastric volume is reduced, the pH can be measured, and more antacid inserted if it is unsatisfactory.

Rout and colleagues used intraoperative gastric emptying to assess the efficacy of intravenous ranitidine (50 mg) given at the time of the decision for caesarean delivery in nearly 600 emergencies requiring general anaesthesia.[7] All women received oral sodium citrate (0.3 M), and either ranitidine or placebo. Those who received ranitidine had a higher pH in all samples; in the citrate only group the trend showed a declining pH with the passage of time with the reverse true in the ranitidine group. After 30 minutes ranitidine was effective in raising pH. This should be adequate when the duration of time from decision to operate to extubation is considered. Rout and colleagues also commented that when gastric contents are particulate, pH is more likely to be unsatisfactory.

It is widely held that the reduction in deaths owing to aspiration is a consequence of prophylaxis with H_2 receptor antagonists.[1] If the number of maternal deaths due to anaesthesia are plotted against the number of caesarean sections performed during successive triennia, three things are apparent. The first is that, from the point of view of mortality as a result of anaesthesia, improvement has ceased. The second is that deaths owing to aspiration and airway problems follow the same pattern, though sometimes

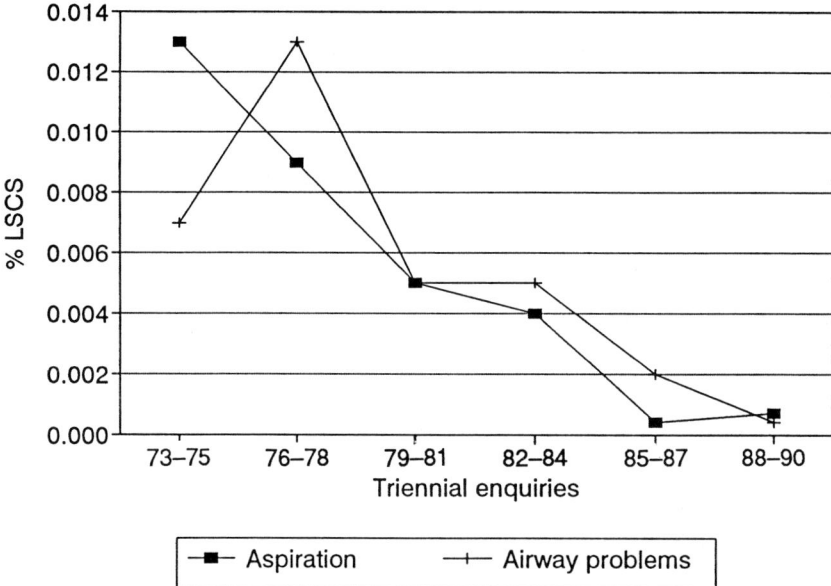

Fig. 4.1   Anaesthetic mortality as a percentage of caesarean sections. Data derived from Reports on Confidential Enquiries into Maternal Deaths in England and Wales 1973–75, 1976–78, 1979–81, 1982–84, and Reports on Confidential Enquiries into Maternal Deaths in the United Kingdom 1985–87, 1988–90, Her Majesty's Stationery Office, London.

the two are inextricably linked.[2] Thirdly, from the early 1970s, when oral antacids were advocated throughout labour for all, to the late 1980s when, in disgrace for their particulate nature, they were replaced by H_2 receptor antagonists, the risk of dying from aspiration at caesarean section plummeted. When H_2 receptor antagonists arrived on the scene, the problem had been largely solved. However, while their importance might be debated, their use with sodium citrate, perhaps in combination with metoclopramide, is not.[8]

An alternative explanation for the decline in maternal mortality is that an increasing number of caesarean sections were being performed using regional anaesthesia. For this to be true we must believe that regional anaesthesia is safer than general anaesthesia, and that the proportional use of general anaesthesia was steadily diminishing over the years studied. Madej and colleagues[9] have shown that, even in the presence of an established epidural service, further reductions in the use of general anaesthesia occur following the introduction of spinal anaesthesia. In particular, their requirement for general anaesthesia for emergency caesarean section fell from 67% to 38%, and the need to rescue regional with general anaesthesia was less common with spinal than with epidural anaesthesia. An opportunity to compare both mortality and morbidity is provided by the North American closed claims experience.[2] Of 1541 closed malpractice claims registered between 1975 and 1985, 190 were obstetric, accounting for 12% of all claims. Of these, 76% were related to anaesthesia, 67% were associated with caesarean delivery, and 33% with general anaesthesia. Anaesthesia for caesarean delivery carries a greater risk of litigation than for non-obstetric procedures. Two claims were made because no anaesthetist was available. The most common damaging events leading to injury related to the respiratory system. Aspiration was cited in 8% of obstetric claims compared with 2% of non-obstetric claims, and half of these were in association with poor airway control and inadequate ventilation. Maternal deaths and events related to the respiratory system were more common with general anaesthesia, while convulsions, headache, backache and pain during anaesthesia were more common with regional. It was judged that 50% of general anaesthetics failed to get the appropriate standard of care compared with 33% of regional. Financial settlement was made in 63% of general anaesthetic claims compared with 48% of regional. Maternal death rate for general anaesthetic claims was 42% compared with 12% for regional.[2] Choice of anaesthesia may be the critical factor in reducing mortality.[8]

Other factors that may imply increased risk include obesity, pre-existing cardiovascular disease, poor facilities for postoperative care,[8] and Asian and Afro Caribbean ethnic origin.[10]

If further decreases in mortality due to anaesthesia are unlikely, attention should be focussed on haemorrhage. If deaths from haemorrhage are combined with deaths from ectopic pregnancy they make up 25% of all maternal deaths in the United Kingdom,[1] but significant haemorrhage during caesarean section is rare. Less than 10% of Caesarean sections require transfusion. When blood loss at elective caesarean section was measured by the alkaline haematin method, mean loss was found to be 487 ml, but the greatest single loss was 1438 ml.[11] A questionnaire study discovered that 87% of units have a blood bank on site, and 82% have a protocol for massive haemorrhage, but only 76% have an intensive care unit to take their survivors.[12] Even when there is a blood bank on site, most do not have a resident technician and are subject to out of hours delays.[13] Further improvements in maternal mortality may require substantial attention to the infrastructure.

GENERAL ANAESTHESIA

King and Colleagues,[14] wishing to assess the adequacy of their general anaesthetic technique for caesarean section, used an isolated arm, a computerized cerebral function monitor, and a tape that played target words and simple instructions repeatedly, on 30 women having elective operations. Each received thiopentone to a maximum dose of 250 mg and suxamethonium (1.5 mg/kg), and the abdominal incision was made immediately after intubation. Anaesthesia was maintained with 0.5% halothane in 50% nitrous oxide, and an infusion of suxamethonium. The majority of patients signalled pain via their isolated arm for the first minute of surgery, and one-third demonstrated signs of awareness at laryngoscopy and intubation. None had recall. They concluded that their anaesthetic was inadequate for the skin incision.[14] This approach to general anaesthesia has become largely historical in the United Kingdom. Awareness can be abolished by increasing the induction dose of thiopentone from 3–4 mg/kg to 5–7 mg/kg and replacing halothane with isoflurane 1%, continued to the end of the operation in a lower concentration. Halothane has fallen from favour because thymol accumulation can interfere with vaporizer output, while isoflurane and enflurance are free of preservative.[15]

Induction agent

For many the choice of induction agent remains thiopentone. A report from Germany comparing thiopentone with ketamine found that the latter was associated with the least drop in blood pressure, and 24% of those given ketamine experienced nightmares.[16] A comparison of thiopentone (5 mg/kg) with propofol (2.4 mg/kg) and midazolam (0.3 mg/kg) showed that midazolam was slow to induce, perhaps increasing risk from aspiration, and in common with propofol, produced doubts about the depth of anaesthesia, and lower Apgar and neurobehavioural scores. The depth of anaesthesia was assessed using the EEG, which is unsuitable for this purpose.[17] Midazolam produces dense amnesia.[18] Concern over awareness with these two drugs is not really justified by the findings. What is of interest is that propofol induction was followed by a significant drop in blood pressure,[19] since blunting of the pressor response to laryngoscopy and intubation continues to preoccupy obstetric anaesthetists. Gin and colleagues[20] studied noradrenaline and adrenaline levels in 61 Chinese women during induction with thiopentone (4 mg/kg) or propofol (2 mg/kg). Propofol was more effective at attenuating the pressor response to intubation, the difference being more marked with noradrenaline than adrenaline. Neonatal assessment included Apgar and neurobehavioural scores, and biochemistry of both umbilical arterial and venous blood. Unlike Celleno's group[19] no neonatal differences were found, perhaps because there was no significant hypotension.[20] An excellent review concluded that no real neonatal or maternal advantages have been demonstrated for propofol over thiopentone for caesarean section,[21] and more recent investigations have not changed this position. It may be that propofol will find a niche in the induction of pre-eclamptics for caesarean section, but an alternative option is to give alfentanil (10 µg/kg) at induction. Dann and colleagues found that this dose, given with thiopentone (3.5 mg/kg), significantly obtunded the pressor response without affecting Apgar scores 10 minutes later.[22] No neurobehavioural assessments were made and uterine to delivery times were absent, but the technique is clinically acceptable.

Ventilation and maintenance

There is general agreement that the physiological carbon dioxide tension of the third trimester, 4 kPa, should be preserved during general anaesthesia. This requires a minute volume of 120 ml/kg of fresh gas before delivery, and 109 ml/kg after.[23] For many years the notion that the inspired oxygen concentration should be 50% has gone unchallenged. Lawes and colleagues were unable to detect any differences in outcome in women receiving either 50% or 33% inspired oxygen in nitrous oxide,[24] and Bogod and colleagues were unconvinced that giving 100% oxygen produced any clinically significant improvement on 50%.[25] However, a general conclusion cannot be extrapolated to any individual hypoxic fetus, especially when each group contained only five emergency caesarean sections.[25] If 100% oxygen is chosen, then either isoflurane or enflurane at 3% for 3 minutes, and then continued at isoflurane 1.25% or enflurane 1.5%, will provide adequate anaesthesia with no awareness, satisfactory uterine contractility, and no undue depression of the fetus.[26] When 0.5% halothane was compared with 0.75% isoflurane, the latter group required less oxytocin, uterine contractility as assessed by the surgeon was better, and mothers recovered more quickly.[27] Awareness has been reported with isoflurane 1% in 50% nitrous oxide[15] so a lower concentration cannot be recommended. Higher arterial concentrations of isoflurane can be achieved by turning up the vaporizer early in the operation and then gradually reducing, rather than using a 1% concentration continuously.[28] Much of this work is already obsolete. A modern anaesthetic machine with integral monitoring, including accurate and reliable gas sampling, will allow an anaesthetist to oxygenate to an optimum saturation, ventilate to a given end expired carbon dioxide tension, and vary vaporizer output to maintain a given end expired tension of volatile agent. This should improve efficacy of general anaesthesia for the mother, minimize factors such as hypocapnia and light anaesthesia that might limit blood flow to the fetus, and probably represents the single most important advance in general obstetric anaesthesia in recent years.

New drugs may well struggle to find a place. A preliminary report suggests that desflurane is satisfactory for caesarean section,[29] comparative studies as yet are unavailable. Vecuronium (0.1 mg/kg) works more quickly in patients undergoing caesarean section than non-pregnant controls with mean onset at 80 seconds and good conditions for intubation; recovery took longer, 46 compared to 28 minutes.[30] The more rapid onset compared with the controls is attributed to increased cardiac output of pregnancy, less protein binding, and relative overdosage. The last point is relevant because water-soluble polar drugs like muscle relaxants do not cross the placenta, and the dose was calculated according to pregnant weight. It would also explain the longer recovery. Teviotdale assessed vecuronium as a substitute for suxamethonium, with thiopentone, in 30 emergency sections, without problem.[31] Abouleish and colleagues assessed rocuronium (0.6 mg/kg) with thiopentone (6 mg/kg) in a significantly more exacting study. Intubating conditions were good or excellent in 90% of patients after waiting 80 seconds.[32] No suxamethonium was used in any of these studies. Teviotdale, in particular, gives as one of his aims the investigation of aspects of clinical safety consequent upon substituting suxamethonium with the longer acting non-depolarizing muscle relaxant. A failed intubation drill in this circumstance cannot depend on abandoning general anaesthesia, and he is taken to task for advocating a technique that puts women at increased risk.[33] One unit's incidence of failed intubation is 1:280 general anaesthetics,[10] and a series of 30 patients is insufficient to realise the aims of the study. As the use of general anaesthesia declines in the Western world, so does the number of potential recruits to research projects.

REGIONAL ANAESTHESIA

Hypotension, preload, vasopressors and neonatal acidosis

Hypotension remains a significant problem with spinal anaesthesia, despite widespread use of volume loading, prompting Rout and colleagues to question the value of preload.[34] In a study of complex design, 78 women received 20 ml/kg of Plasmalyte with their spinal anaesthetic and 62 did not. Hypotension was defined as systolic pressure lower than 100 mmHg, or a reduction to 80% of baseline. Fifty-five per cent of the preload group were hypotensive compared with 71% of the abstainers. While this reaches statistical significance, analysis reveals that over 50% of both groups were hypotensive, and against this figure an intergroup difference of 16% is of lesser importance. If only 16% benefit from preload, it can hardly be considered a vital part of the procedure.[34] In another study the same group investigated the effects of giving the preload over 10 minutes instead of 20.[35] They found that the incidence of hypotension was the same in both groups, and that fast infusion produced some worrying high central venous pressures. The next step was to compare crystalloid preload with an infusion of ephedrine. Gajraj and colleagues chose to test this on 54 women undergoing post partum sterilizations. Half received 15 ml/kg of Ringer's lactate, and half received ephedrine (50 mg in 50 ml) via a syringe pump, titrating the infusion rate against the blood pressure, once primed. A standard spinal anaesthetic was performed on all. The preload group experienced the same incidence of hypotension as Rout and colleagues, 55%, but the incidence of hypotension in the ephedrine group was 22%. Prophylactic administration of vasopressor is associated with larger overall doses than when given as required, and nausea and vomiting still occurs. The degree of hypotension in this study was mild compared to that sometimes found in pregnant patients who are liable to aortocaval compression.[36] If the case against preload is accepted, then prophylactic vasopressor must become routine, and recommendations are required with regard to choice of drug and route of administration, taking into account effects on uteroplacental flow. One technique not to be recommended is the use of intramuscular (IM) ephedrine. Approximately 4% of all spinal anaesthetics fail, many requiring general anaesthesia, and the combination of general anaesthesia and vasopressor may be a source of neonatal acidosis. Babies born following the administration of 50 mg ephedrine (IM) and a general anaesthetic were significantly more acidotic than controls. Effects of 25 mg were less marked, but it failed to work in 50% of cases.[37]

There are two techniques used to study maternal circulation during caesarean section. Cardiac output can be measured noninvasively using either Doppler echocardiography, or thoracic electrical bioimpedance. The latter has only recently become available to clinical anaesthetists as a monitor that measures the resistance of the thorax to the flow of a high frequency, constant, and low magnitude alternating current that is imperceptible to the subject under study. Measurement produces a steady-state component and a pulsatile component. The steady-state component is called the Thoracic Fluid Index and reflects the volume of intrathoracic fluids. The pulsatile components are computer processed to generate cardiac output, ejection fraction, and end-diastolic volume. All this requires is two pairs of electrodes at the root of the neck and at the diaphragm. The normal pattern during epidural anaesthesia is for the cardiac index to rise from baseline to reach its highest value at delivery, aided to a major extent by an increase in heart rate. Ejection fraction rises only slightly from baseline, but the increase is maintained to the end of the operation. End diastolic volume is an index of heart filling, and so it rises with volume loading, but by the end of surgery has settled to baseline values.[38] The uteroplacental circulation is assessed using Doppler probes aimed at vessels on either side of the placenta, and in more sophisticated studies the fetal cerebral and renal circulations will also be scrutinized. Rising Doppler pulsatility index implies increasing vascular resistance and reduced flow. Cardiac output may be a more important factor in the maintenance of the fetal circulation than arterial pressure. Robson and colleagues[39] used Doppler echocardiography to compare the maternal and fetal haemodynamic changes during elective spinal and epidural anaesthesia. They found that vascular resistance in the fetal umbilical placental bed was greater with spinal anaesthesia, and that there was a correlation between maternal cardiac output, umbilical artery pH and umbilical artery pulsatility index, and concluded that cardiac output was a better predictor of uteroplacental function than arterial pressure. A few of the neonates in the spinal arm of this study were sufficiently acidotic to bring spinal anaesthesia into question. It should be pointed out that despite using an ephedrine infusion, more than 50% of the patients receiving anaesthesia in this study were hypotensive,[39] suggesting that the infusion was ineffective. Hypotension can be avoided if the ephedrine is infused briskly at the onset of spinal anaesthesia, and when this has been done efficiently, neonatal acidosis does not occur.[40] Umbilical arterial base excess is lower following an episode of hypotension,[34] and an infusion of vasopressor is better than bolus administration.[41] Valli and colleagues[42] investigated the effects of epidural, spinal, and a combined epidural/spinal anaesthesia on uteroplacental pulsatility indices. The combined technique used involved a spinal for the lower half of the block and epidural for the upper half. Etilefrine, an alpha and beta agonist, was infused. In the spinal group alone there was an increase in vascular resistance in the uterine artery, but no difference in any fetal parameters were found. They concluded that the changes with spinal anaesthesia were not of clinical importance.[42] The commonest vasopressor used in caesarean section is ephedrine, which has combined alpha and beta actions, but recently pure alpha agonists have been in vogue. One advantage of the pure alpha agonist should be less disturbance in heart rate. Wright and colleagues[43] compared ephedrine with the alpha agonist methoxamine to treat hypotension during elective epidural anaesthesia, using equipotent doses as required. Both drugs were effective at controlling hypotension, but methoxamine produced significant increases in fetal and maternal heart rates, and increased vascular resistance on the maternal side of the placenta. Ephedrine was innocuous, and methoxamine was not recommended. What is important here is that hypotension was also associated with an increase in uterine vascular resistance, but unlike changes due to the vasopressor the flow resistance persisted. In women who remained normotensive, flow resistance reduced slightly once the block had become established. Placental pH gradients were therefore greater after an episode of hypotension when compared with normotensives.[43] Unravelling this for the clinical anaesthetist, the message is clear. When hypotension occurs with spinal anaesthesia, it may be associated with an unpredictable degree of neonatal acidosis. This can be prevented by a prophylactic administration of vasopressor that must be infused sufficiently rapidly to be effective when maximal hypotension occurs around the 6th or 7th minute. Ephedrine remains the vasopressor of choice, but whereas undesirable effects of vasopressors are transient, those caused by hypotension may not be. When spinal anaesthesia is performed with appropriate attention to detail, the neonatal outcome is the same as that following epidural anaesthesia, but inexpert spinal anaesthesia may be inferior to any adequate form of epidural anaesthesia.

Emergency anaesthesia and neonatal outcome

The arguments above are only valid for elective surgery. In the emergency situation, effective existing epidural blocks should be extended otherwise the time factor necessitates a choice between spinal and general anaesthesia. Prospective comparisons between spinal and general anaesthesia are difficult because maternal choice can influence randomization, and careful attention to detail is required to optimize neonatal condition. Accepting these limitations, Hodgson and Wauchob[44] found a greater degree of neonatal acidosis, following general as opposed to spinal anaesthesia, in 137 women undergoing elective surgery. Ephedrine was given as required to the spinal group. Apgar scores are generally unhelpful since neonates subjected to general anaesthesia require a recovery period and airway support for a short time. Consequently they score poorly initially, but this does not necessarily imply an adverse prognosis. A comparison of Apgar scores of 509 singleton premature babies (gestational age less than 32 weeks), born by caesarean section with either general or epidural anaesthesia, found that after general anaesthesia, 46% scored three or less at 1 minute, whereas after epidural the figure was 22%. The authors argued that in this situation, the 1 minute Apgar score identified infants in need of cardiopulmonary resuscitation (CPR), and the 5 minute score reflected the outcome of CPR. After 5 minutes, 10% still had scores of three or less, compared with 4% after epidural. Anaesthetic techniques were not standardized, and indications for choice of anaesthesia were unknown. It may be that, when choice of anaesthesia for small babies exists, it should be for epidural.[45]

Epidural anaesthesia

Lignocaine 2% with adrenaline 1 in 200 000 has become a popular choice for caesarean section because it combines relatively rapid onset time with dense block. The adrenaline is necessary because therapeutic volumes of 2% lignocaine for epidural anaesthesia can produce systemic effects in mother and baby. It also prolongs the action. Perhaps because of the history of spinal anaesthesia in the United Kingdom, there is more of a reluctance to use a vasoconstrictor in this site than there is in North America. The main concern stems from the singularity of the blood supply to the cord, and its vulnerability to vasoconstrictor–induced ischaemia. Loss of the anterior spinal artery will produce paraplegia. It may be that the risk is theoretical, and that the clinical advantages justify its use.[46] Alahuta and colleagues[47] were concerned that epidural adrenaline might have adverse effects on the circulation of the compromised fetus. They studied 23 women, with gestational ages between 28 and 36 weeks, requiring caesarean section for pregnancy induced hypertension. Some of the women were taking labetalol, but the groups were balanced. Half received plain bupivacaine, and half bupivacaine with adrenaline. They found an increase in flow resistance in the uteroplacental vessels following adrenaline. This was accompanied by a decrease in flow resistance in the fetal renal and cerebral circulations. There were no differences in neonatal biochemistry between the groups. Their two postulates were that the fetus was autoregulating in the face of reduced perfusion, and that adrenaline might have exerted a direct effect. It is too soon to say that adrenaline is innocuous to the compromised fetus.

Fentanyl

The use of epidural fentanyl improves the quality of intraoperative analgesia. When 50 µg is compared with 100 µg, the only difference between the two is that the higher dose produces more pruritus,[48] whilst 50 µg is no better than 25 µg.[49] Breen and Janzen[50] investigated whether fentanyl given after delivery worked as well as a dose given before. When they found no difference they concluded that it was better from the baby's point of view for it to be given after delivery. While the logic of this is debatable, perusal of their data should be sufficient to convince any potential patient and most anaesthetists that fentanyl is best given before surgery.[50]

Alkalinization and warming

Alkalinization of local anaesthetic to bring pH closer to pKa (7.9 for lignocaine), should render more of the unionized moiety available to diffuse through tissues. When bicarbonate has been added to achieve this, its breakdown, hopefully at the axon, will produce CO_2, reducing pH and promoting ionization, so that the ionized moiety can block conduction. It is also possible that CO_2 may have a direct action on calcium channels. Alkalinization of epidural local anaesthetics is known to improve intraoperative comfort, but is there any advantage if fentanyl is used? Capogna and colleagues[51] investigated lignocaine 2% with adrenaline and fentanyl 100 µg at pH 6.575 and pH 7.138. There was no difference in onset time to T4, but the alkalinized group required less supplements. Maternal plasma and umbilical artery levels of fentanyl were higher, so improved analgesia might have been due to increased systemic absorption. This requires further testing with smaller doses of fentanyl.

Reduction in onset time of 3 minutes can be achieved by warming the lignocaine to 38°C, and it beats bupivacaine at room temperature by 5 minutes.[52]

Spinal anaesthesia

The rationale for adding adrenaline to intrathecal local anaesthetics is less distinct than with epidural. Effects on systemic absorption are of no clinical significance, and duration of anaesthesia is not usefully increased.[53] Adding 100 µg or 200 µg adrenaline to intrathecal bupivacaine can reduce the mean time to T4 by 2 minutes,[54] but this does not impress. The addition of fentanyl (0.25 µg/kg) to intrathecal bupivacaine reduces the need for supplements during surgery without adverse effects, and provides 4 to 5 hours postoperative comfort. Increasing doses produce sleepier patients, slower regression to T12, and longer postoperative comfort.[55] Abouleish and colleagues claim that best intraoperative comfort can be achieved by adding both adrenaline (200 µg) and morphine (200 µg) to intrathecal bupivacaine. They postulate that the improved analgesia is due to a direct effect on adrenergic receptors in the cord.[56]

Pethidine is an opioid analgesic with local anaesthetic effects: 1 mg/kg of a 5% solution (specific gravity 1.026), when given intrathecally, will produce a block that lasts in the region of 1 hour. Compared with 5% hyperbaric lignocaine, onset time is slightly slower, block height slightly lower with less motor blockade, more pruritus, but less hypotension and up to 6 hours postoperative comfort.[57] This may be useful when conventional techniques are contraindicated, but information regarding respiratory depression is required.

A useful practical tip to speed an adequate block height when using a combined spinal/epidural technique, is to inject a fluid bolus epidurally. This is a volume effect that shifts the intrathecal anaesthetic cephalad.[58] If epidural local anaesthetic is used both techniques are supported.

Chest pain, air embolism and ECG changes

Referred pain from nociceptive afferents in the parietal peritoneum can give rise to chest pain during surgery.[59] Doppler probes detected air embolism in 4% to 52% of Caesarean sections,[60] and electrocardiogram (ECG) monitoring showed definite ST segment depression in 30% to 60%.[61] The temptation to link these three unconnected findings is hard to resist. Expired nitrogen measurement is more sensitive than Doppler, and its use confirms that air embolism occurs during most Caesarean sections, usually in association with the open uterus.[60] Enzyme assays and echocardiography have failed to find evidence of myocardial ischaemia, and cardiac sympathetic block is being considered as a possible cause of ST segment depression.[61] The occurrence of chest pain continues to have clinical significance and requires treatment as before.

POSTOPERATIVE ANALGESIA

Non steroidal anti-inflammatory drugs (NSAIDs)

The morphine sparing effects of NSAIDs, demonstrated with other forms of surgery, occurs after caesarean section. Diclofenac (75 mg) intramuscularly after general anaesthesia or 100 mg rectally after spinal anaesthesia augments intravenous morphine analgesia with a patient-controlled analgesia system (PCAS).[62,63] When used in combination with epidural morphine, patient satisfaction is improved and rescue analgesia is not required.[64] Side-effects of morphine are unaffected. NSAIDs are contraindicated in pre-eclampsia, but choice of drug does not appear to be important.[65] Quantities of diclofenac in breast milk are negligible,[62] and patient acceptability is high.

Patient controlled epidural analgesia (PCEAS)

Epidural opioids can provide the best analgesia, but PCAS score highest on patient satisfaction. PCEAS might provide the best of both worlds. Yu and Gambling compared epidural morphine (3 mg) with fentanyl by PCEAS.[66] Satisfaction was the same in both groups, but the PCEAS patients used significantly more fentanyl, and the morphine group had more pruritus. Both groups had subclinical respiratory depression when measured at 4 and 8 hours. When compared with intravenous PCAS, PCEAS achieved similar pain and sedation scores, but patients used less opioid, were taking solid food earlier and were ready for discharge sooner.[67] Not all patients are enthusiastic about keeping their epidural catheter, and if it migrates out analgesia fails.[66] It remains to be seen if PCEAS will become an established technique.

Intrathecal morphine

Doses of preservative-free intrathecal morphine (100 to 200 µg) can provide effective analgesia for over 24 hours.[68] Doses as low as 80 µg are more effective than an oral regimen of morphine sulphate tablets.[69] Even with minute doses, nausea, vomiting and pruritus can be troublesome.

Clonidine

Clonidine is an alpha-2 adrenergic agonist that can exert anti-nociceptive effects via receptors in the dorsal cord. When 150 µg is given intrathecally, analgesia comes on in 10 minutes, and the best pain relief occurs 90 minutes after injection. Duration is 4 to 12 hours.[70] The same dose given epidurally has an onset time of 15 minutes and lasts 2 to 5 hours. Use of clonidine is associated with hypotension and sedation, and it has failed to gain a foothold.[71]

KEY POINTS FOR CLINICAL PRACTICE

- Mortality as a result of anaesthesia is no longer falling.
- Haemorrhage is responsible for 25% of all maternal deaths.
- Awareness during caesarean section under general anaesthesia can be abolished by giving thiopentone 5–7 mg/kg, and isoflurane 1%, continued after delivery at a lesser concentration.
- Volume loading is inferior to prophylactic vasopressor in avoiding hypotension during regional anaesthesia.
- Ephedrine remains the vasopressor of choice.
- Hypotension associated with spinal anaesthesia may be responsible for a degree of neonatal acidosis.
- Epidural anaesthesia may be the best choice for the compromised fetus.

- NSAIDs are a useful adjunct to postoperative analgesic regimens.
- A single dose of intrathecal morphine (100 μg to 200 μg) provides long lasting analgesia, but is associated with nausea, vomiting and pruritus.
- Spinal clonidine has analgesic properties, but is associated with sedation and hypotension.

REFERENCES

1. Department of Health. Report on Confidential Enquiries into Maternal Deaths in the United Kingdom. Her Majesty's Stationery Office, London, 1994
2. Chadwick H S, Posner K, Caplan R et al. A comparison of obstetric and non obstetric anesthesia malpractice claims. Anesthesiology 1991; 74: 242–249
3. Treffers P E, Pel M. The rising trend for caesarean birth. BMJ 1993; 307: 1017–1018
4. James C. Litigation and caesarean section. J Med Defence Union 1993; 4: 78
5. Leitch C R, Walker J J. Caesarean section rates. BMJ 1994; 308: 133
6. May A E. The confidential enquiry into maternal deaths 1988–90. Br J Anaesth 1994; 73: 129–131
7. Rout C C, Rocke D A, Gouws E. Intravenous ranitidine reduces the risk of acid aspiration of gastric contents at emergency caesarean section. Anesth Analg 1993; 76: 156–161
8. Thomas T A. Maternal mortality. Int J Obst Anaesth 1994; 3: 125–126
9. Madej T H, Jackson I B, Wheatley R G, Wilson J. Assessing introduction of spinal anaesthesia for obstetric procedures. Quality in Health Care 1993; 2: 31–34
10. Bonney G, Lyons G. Failed intubation drill: A review of its use in obstetric practice. Int J Obstet Anaesth 1994; 3: 108
11. Duthie S J, Ghosh A, Ng A, Ho P C. Intraoperative blood loss during elective lower segment caesarean section. Br J Obstet Gynaecol 1992; 99: 364–367
12. Hibbard B, Milner D. Reports on confidential enquiries into maternal deaths: An audit of previous recommendations. Health Trends 1994; 26: 26–28
13. Clark V A, Wardall G J, McGrady E M. Blood ordering practices in obstetric units in the United Kingdom. Anaesthesia 1993; 48: 998–1007
14. King H, Ashley S, Braithwaite D et al. Adequacy of general anesthesia for caesarean section. Anesth Analg 1993; 77: 84–88
15. Lyons G, Macdonald R. Awareness during caesarean section. Anaesthesia 1991; 46: 62–64
16. Krissel J, Dick W F, Leyser K H et al. Thiopentone, thiopentone/ketamine and ketamine for induction of anaesthesia in caesarean section. Eur J Anaesthesiol 1994; 11: 115–122
17. Hanning C D, Aitkenhead A R. Sleep, depth of anaesthesia and awareness. In: Nimmo W S, Rowbotham D J, Smith G (eds) Anaesthesia 2nd edn. Blackwell, Oxford, 1994
18. Reilly C S. Intravenous anaesthetic agents. In: Nimmo W S, Rowbotham D J, Smith G (eds) Anaesthesia 2nd edn. Blackwell, Oxford, 1994
19. Celleno D, Capogna G, Emmanuelli M et al. Which induction agent for cesarean section? A comparison of thiopentone sodium, propofol and midazolam. J Clin Anaesth 1993; 5: 284–288
20. Gin T, O'Meara M E, Kan A F et al. Plasma catecholamines and neonatal condition after induction of anaesthesia with propofol or thiopentone at caesarean section. Br J Anaesth 1993; 70: 311–316
21. Capogna G, Celleno D. Effects on the baby of maternal analgesia and anaesthesia. In: Reynolds F (ed) The effects of anaesthetic agents on the newborn, W B Saunders, London, 1993
22. Dann W L, Hutchinson A, Cartwright D P. Maternal and neonatal responses to alfentanil administered before induction of general anaesthesia for caesarean section. Br J Anaesth 1987; 59: 1392–1396

23. Rampton A J, Malliah S, Garrett C P. Increased ventilation requirements during obstetrical general anaesthesia. Br J Anaesth 1988; 61: 730–737
24. Lawes E G, Newman B, Campbell M J et al. Maternal inspired oxygen concentration and neonatal status for caesarean section under general anaesthesia. Br J Anaesth 1988; 61: 250–254
25. Bogod D G, Rosen M, Rees G A D. Maximum FIO$_2$ during caesarean section. Br J Anaesth 1988; 61: 255–262
26. Tunstall M E, Sheik A. Comparison of 1.5% enflurane with 1.25% isoflurane in oxygen for caesarean section: avoidance of awareness without nitrous oxide. Br J Anaesth 1989; 62: 138–143
27. Ghaly R G, Flynn R J. Isoflurane as an alternative to halothane for caesarean section. Anaesthesia 1988; 43: 5–7
28. McCrirrick A, Evans G H, Thomas T A. Overpressure of isoflurane at caesarean section: a study of areterial isoflurane concentrations. Br J Anaesth 1994; 72: 122–124
29. Whitten C W, Elmore J C, Larson T W. Desflurane: a review. Progress in Anesthesiology 1993; 7: 54
30. Baraka A, Jabbour S, Tabboush Z. et al. Onset of vecuronium neuromuscular block is more rapid in patients underoging caesarean section. Can J Anaesth 1992; 39: 135–138
31. Teviotdale B M. Vecuronium – thiopentone induction for emergency caesarean section under general anaesthesia. Anaesth Intens Care 1993; 21: 288–291
32. Abouleish E, Abboud T, Lechevalier T et al. Rocuronium for caesarean section. Br J Anaesth 1994; 73: 336–341
33. Brimacombe J, Berry A. Vecuronium for emergency caesarean section. Anaesth Intens Care 1994; 22: 119–120
34. Rout C C, Rocke D A, Levin J et al. A re-evaluation of the role of crystalloid preload in the prevention of hypotension associated with spinal anesthesia for elective cesarean section. Anesthesiology 1993; 79: 262–269
35. Rout C C, Akoojee S S, Rocke D A, Gouws E. Rapid administration of crystalloid preload does not decrease the incidence of hypotension after spinal anaesthesia for elective caesarean section. Br J Anaesth 1992; 68: 394–397
36. Gajraj N M, Victory R A, Pace N A et al. Comparison of an ephedrine infusion with crystalloid administration for prevention of hypotension during spinal anesthesia. Anesth Analg 1993; 76: 1023–1026
37. Rout C C, Rocke D A, Brijball R, Koovarjee V. Prophylactic intramuscular ephedrine prior to caesarean section. Anaesth Intens Care 1992; 20: 448–452
38. Croby E T, Bryson G L, Elliott R D, Gverzdys C. Epidural sufentanil does not attenuate the central haemodynamic effects of caesarean section performed under epidural anesthesia. Can J Anaesth 1994; 41: 192–197
39. Robson S C, Boys R J, Rodeck C, Morgan B. Maternal and fetal haemodynamic effects of spinal and extradural anaesthesia for elective caesarean section. Br J Anaesth 1992; 68: 54–59
40. Patel M, Swami A, Dent H. Maternal and fetal haemodynamic effects of spinal and extradural anaesthesia for elective caesarean section. Br J Anaesth 1992; 68: 635–636
41. Kang Y G, Abouleish E, Caritis S. Prophylactic intravenous ephedrine infusion during spinal anesthesia for cesarean section. Anesth Analg 1982; 61: 839–842
42. Valli J, Pirhonen J, Aantaa R et al. The effects of regional anaesthesia for caesarean section on maternal and foetal blood flow velocities measured by doppler ultrasound. Acta Anaesthesiol Scand 1994; 38: 1159–
43. Wright P M C, Iftikhar M, Fitzpatrick K T et al. Vasopressor therapy for hypotension during epidural anesthesia for cesarean section: effects on maternal and fetal flow velocity rates. Anesth Analg 1992; 75: 56–63
44. Hodgson C A, Wauchob T D. A comparison of spinal and general anaesthesia for elective caesarean section: effect on neonatal condition at birth. Int J Obstet Anaesth 1994; 3: 25–30
45. Rolbin S H, Cohen M M, Levinton C M et al. The premature infant: anesthesia for cesarean delivery. Anesth Analg 1994; 78: 912–917
46. Moore J K, Hughes S C. There is no place for adrenaline in the epidural or subarachnoid space. Int J Obstet Anaesth 1994; 3: 54–58

47. Alahuta S, Rasanen J, Jouppila P et al. Uteroplacental and fetal circulation during extradural bupivacaine – adrenaline and bupivacaine for caesarean section in hypertensive pregnancies with chronic fetal asphyxia. Br J Anaesth 1993; 71: 348–353
48. Halonen P M, Paatero H. Hovorka J et al. Comparison of two fentanyl doses to improve epidural anaesthesia with 0.5% bupivacaine for caesarean section. Acta Anaesthesiol Scand 1993; 37: 774–779
49. Yee I, Carstoniu J, Halpern S, Pittini R. A comparison of two doses of epidural fentanyl during caesarean section. Can J Anaesth 1993; 40: 722–725
50. Breen, T W, Janzen J A. Epidural fentanyl and caesarean section: when should fentanyl be given? Can J Anaesth 1992; 39: 317–322
51. Capogna G, Celleno D, Costantino P et al. Alkalinisation improves the quality of lidocaine-fentanyl epidural anaesthesia for caesarean section. Can J Anaesth 1993; 40: 425–430
52. Clark V, McGardy E, Sugden C et al. Speed of onset of sensory block of elective extradural caesarean section: choice of agent and temperature of injectate. Br J Anaesth 1994; 72: 221–233
53. Zakowski M I, Ramanatham S, Sharnick S, Turndorf H. Uptake and distribution of bupivacaine and morphine after intrathecal administration in parturients: effects of epinephrine. Anesth Analg 1992; 74: 664–669
54. Moore C H, Wilhite A, Pan P H, Blass N H. The addition of epinephrine to subarachnoid administered hyperbaric bupivacaine with fentanyl for cesarean delivery. Regional Anesth 1992; 17: 202–204
55. Belzarena S D. Clinical effects of intrathecally administered fentanyl in patients undergoing cesarean section. Anesth Analg 1992; 74: 653–657
56. Abouleish E, Rawal N, Tolson-Randall B et al. A clinical and laboratory study to compare the additon of 0.2 mg morphine, 0.2 mg epinephrine, or their combination to hypobaric bupivacaine for spinal anesthesia in cesarean section. Anesth Analg 1993; 77: 457–462
57. Kafle S K. Intrathecal meperidine for elective caesarean section: a comparison with lidocaine. Can J Anaesth 1993; 40: 718–721
58. Blumgart C H, Ryall D, Dennison B, Thompson-Hill M. Mechanism of extension of spina anaesthesia by extradural injection of local anaesthetic. Br J Anaesth 1992; 69: 457–460
59. Palmer C M, Norris M C, Giudici M C et al. Incidence of electrocardiographic changes during cesarean delivery under regional anesthesia. Anesth Analg 1990; 70: 36–43
60. Lew T W K, Tay D H, Thomas E. Venous air embolism during cesarean section: more common than previously thought. Anesth Analg 1993; 77: 448–452
61. Eisenach J C, Tuttle R, Stein A. Is ST segment depression of the electrocardiogram during cesarean section merely due to cardiac sympathetic block? Anesth Analg 1993; 78: 287–292
62. Bush D J, Lyons G, Madonald R. Diclofenac for analgesia after caesarean section. Anaesthesia 1992; 47: 1075–1077
63. Luthman J, Kay N H, White J B. The morphine sparing effect of diclofenac sodium following caesarean section. Int J Obstet Anaesth 1994; 3: 82–86
64. Sun H-L, Wu C-C, Liu M-S et al. Combination of low dose epidural morphine and intramuscular diclofenac sodium in post cesarean analgesia. Anesth Analg 1992; 75: 64–68
65. Rorarius M G F, Suominen P, Baer G A et al. Diclofenac and ketoprofen of pain treatment after caesarean section. Br J Anaesth 1993; 70: 293–297
66. Yu P Y H, Gambling D R. A comparative study of patient controlled epidural fentanyl and single dose epidural morphine for post caesarean analgesia. Can J Anaesth 1993; 40: 416–420
67. Parker R K, White P F. Epidural patient controlled analgesia: an alternative to intravenous patient controlled analgesia for pain relief after cesarean delivery. Anesth Analg 1992; 75: 245–251
68. Uchiyama A, Ueyama H, Nakano S et al. Low dose intrathecal morphine and pain after caesarean section. Int J Obstet Anaesth 1994; 3: 87–91
69. Sibilla C, Abertazzi P, Zatelli R et al. Pain relief after caesarean section: a comparison of different techniques of morphine administration. Int J Obstet Anaesth 1994; 3: 203–207
70. Filos K S, Goudas L C, Patroni O, Polyzou V. Intrathecal clonidine as a sole analgesic for pain relief after cesarean section. Anesthesiology 1992; 77: 267–274
71. Narchi P, Benham D, Hamza J, Bonaziz H. Ventilatory effects of epidural clonidine during the first three hours after caesarean section. Acta Anaesthesiol Scand 1992; 36: 791–795

5

Fibreoptic intubation

A. C. Pearce

Fibreoptic tracheal intubation was first described by Dr Peter Murphy, an anaesthetic Senior Registrar, in 1967.[1] He had read an article in *The Lancet* about the surgical use of a fibreoptic choledochoscope. Much to his surprise, a request to the American manufacturer of this instrument was met by the speedy loan of this new device, which he then used to intubate patients at The National Hospital for Nervous Diseases, Queen's Square, London. The scope did not have a controllable tip and had a side-viewing lens. Subsequent to the initial publication, Murphy had 'hundreds' of requests for reprints from otolaryngologists but not a single anaesthetist asked for information.[2] Over 25 years later, the specialty still seems reluctant to embrace comprehensively the benefits of fibreoptic intubation despite the availability of flexible and rigid fibrescopes specifically designed for anaesthetic use. Generally accepted indications for the use of a flexible fibrescope are given in Table 5.1.

TRAINING

The percentage of consultant anaesthetists who are competent at fibreoptic intubation in the UK remains low. A study from the North of England gauged competency rates by asking the College Tutor at each of 29 hospital departments to estimate the percentage of trained consultants at their own

Table 5.1 Indications for use of intubating fibrescope

Difficult intubation

Awake intubation
- prior to patient positioning (e.g. prone)
- ? cervical spine trauma

Correct placement of:
- double lumen tubes
- single lumen tubes
- nasopharyngeal airway

Changing tracheal tubes
Trial of extubation
Upper airway endoscopy
Lower airway endoscopy

hospital.[3] The average was 28%, with a range of 0–80%. Half of the proficient consultants worked in teaching hospitals. Virtually all hospitals had an intubating fibrescope and the KeyMed company confirm that nationally all acute units possess at least one flexible fibrescope.

Two recent editorials have addressed the issues surrounding training.[4,5] The 'fibre scopes are expensive and a department may possess only one. They are relatively easy to damage, limiting unsupervized use. A situation found commonly in a department is the presence of one or two trained consultants who attempt to teach senior trainees. The trainees leave the department at regular intervals and there remains no critical mass of trained practitioners within the department; teacher fatigue ensues. Training programmes have been formally evaluated and appear to be effective.[6] Commonly, novices gain manipulative skills on models and then progress to patients. Workshops with models only can be partly effective; in one study 35% of attendees were able subsequently to introduce fibreoptic intubation into their clinical practice or improve their success rate.[7] Video facilities allow display of the view through the fibrescope to be projected onto a screen. Both trainee and teacher see the same view, which may be recorded for later discussion, and this significantly increases the efficacy of teaching.[8]

TECHNIQUES

Patients may be intubated orally or nasally, awake or anaesthetised (asleep).

Asleep

Asleep techniques offer considerable advantages and disadvantages. These methods are suitable in any patient in whom it is possible to inflate the lungs easily when anaesthetised using a facemask, provided there is no increased risk of aspiration. It is essential, in introductory teaching cases, that spontaneous or controlled ventilation is continued during the intubation procedure so that oxygen and inhalational anaesthesia (if required) are given continuously. Asleep techniques have the advantages that the patient and trainee are not made uncomfortable by the intubation procedure and can be used also by anaesthetists to maintain their skills during normal operating lists. The disadvantages are that the oropharyngeal 'space' tends to diminish and must be maintained by jaw thrust, and anaesthesia/ventilation issues must be addressed simultaneously with fibreoptic intubation: two anaesthetists, or an anaesthetist and trained assistant, are essential.

In all techniques, consideration must be given to abolition of laryngeal reflexes. This may be achieved by deep anaesthesia, or by using suxamethonium once the larynx has been identified, before trying to pass the instrument through the vocal cords. Alternatively, this may be achieved by muscle relaxation, using non-depolarizing agents given at the onset of anaesthesia. The abolition of laryngeal reflexes by deep inhalational anaesthesia is fraught with difficulties and this method cannot be recommended for routine use. Calder's group[9] give an honest appraisal of a technique of nasotracheal intubation under oxygen-nitrous oxide-halothane anaesthesia with topical 4% lignocaine sprayed on to the larynx via the fibrescope. The incidence of hypotension and hypoxaemia was alarming, with one patient testing the lower range of oximeter function (18%). In several patients coughing occurred either after airway insertion or on application of lignocaine to the cords. In other patients, cardiovascular depression ensued. There is little rationale to the routine use of a spontaneously breathing, deep inhalational technique for asleep fibreoptic intubation; if the airway is – or is likely to be – difficult to manage, the patient should be intubated awake or an alternative route of ventilation established before induction of anaesthesia.

Laryngeal mask. A laryngeal mask is inserted and the fibrescope introduced through the lumen.[10] The size of tracheal tube that may be used is restricted to 6 mm and the laryngeal mask can be removed only with temporary removal of the tracheal tube connector. The technical difficulty of removing the laryngeal mask over the tracheal tube can be eased by using a second tracheal tube[11] or long plastic tube[12] as a blocker. The split laryngeal mask[13] is a particularly useful modification and allows easy removal of the mask from the fibrescope and selection of any size of tracheal tube. A technique that has been described for teaching, and to allow nasal intubation, is withdrawal of a correctly placed laryngeal mask into the oropharynx (to provide a route for ventilation) with nasotracheal fibreoptic intubation.[14] A laryngeal mask can be inserted in an awake patient under topical anaesthesia.[15]

Oral/Nasal airway. Ventilation is carried out through an oral or nasal airway whilst fibreoptic intubation is undertaken via the unoccupied orifice. The oral tower airway is useful and effective.[16] This technique was first described using a spontaneous breathing technique (halothane), with suxamethonium administration after laryngeal identification, but is probably more often used now with full muscle relaxation throughout. This avoids the problem that occurs if the trainee touches the vocal cords unexpectedly before muscle relaxants have been administered. A dedicated nasopharyngeal airway for ventilation permits both oral and nasotracheal fibreoptic intubation.[17] Nasopharyngeal airway insertion does not appear to give rise to bacteraemia.[18] It is possible to use a small facemask over the mouth, leaving the nose clear for intubation.[19]

Modified facemask/breathing circuit connector. Fibre-endoscopy can be undertaken via small holes in the facemask or breathing circuit connector. The difficulty arises in trying to design a diaphragm that will produce a seal around the fibrescope alone (4 mm) and will enlarge to accommodate a tracheal tube. Diaphragm rupture may allow small particles to enter the patient's airway.[20] The Mainz universal adaptor (Rusch UK) can be fitted with replacement sealing caps.

No airway control simultaneously with intubation. A spontaneously breathing technique[21] involving thiopentone, with supplemental oxygen supplied near the mouth, has been described after long usage in one hospital with great success; muscle paralysis is initiated after identification of the vocal cords. More commonly, an apnoeic technique is used for endoscopy and intubation.[22] One such might be described:

Preoxygenation—propofol/opioid—muscle relaxation—facemask ventilation with oxygen and anaesthesia with supplemental propofol— mask removal —intubation via nose or mouth

This technique is extremely useful for routine difficult intubation and teaching of all but novices. It is not useful for new trainees or in difficult fibreoptic intubations because ventilation is not conducted simultaneously with intubation – if hypoxaemia intervenes, the fibrescope must be withdrawn to allow further mask ventilation. However, 100% oxygen administration allows several minutes of safe apnoea and the intubation is unencumbered by requirements for special equipment. This technique is particularly useful because it allows anaesthetists to maintain their skills on routine patient lists. The retention of learned skills by regular practice is essential and is not emphasized sufficiently in training programmes.

Awake

Fibreoptic intubation is accomplished following topical anaesthesia of the airway. Patients remain conscious, maintain their own airways and are able to help the endoscopist by voluntary cord movement at appropriate moments. In difficult cases, positional changes from lying to sitting are easily accomplished. Mason[4] extols the advantages of trainees learning on awake patients on respiratory physicians' bronchoscopy lists.

The superb article by Benumof[23] gives details of techniques for awake tracheal intubation (by all possible devices); other articles give comprehensive advice for awake fibreoptic intubation[24] and describe one technique in detail,[25] with validation in patients. Awake intubation video recordings are available from KeyMed and Rusch. Nasotracheal awake intubation carries certain advantages. The route to the larynx is often easier than via the mouth, and the patient is unable to bite the fibrescope. It may be contraindicated by surgical demands, nasal pathology or bleeding disorders. The nasal mucosa is anaesthetised/vasoconstricted by topical cocaine 5% (2–3 ml) or a mixture of lignocaine 4% with xylometazoline 0.05%.

The larynx can be anaesthetised directly by topical 4% lignocaine (3– 4 ml) sprayed down the suction channel directly on to the cords (spray-as-you-go) or by injection of the same volume via cricothyroid puncture. In the spray-as-you-go technique, tracheal anaesthesia can be obtained by another 4 ml of 4% lignocaine injected through the suction channel into the trachea. Performance of a transtracheal injection of local anaesthetic prior to endoscopy ensures that the larynx and trachea are anaesthetised and unresponsive when reached with the fibrescope. The risks of transtracheal injection are small (but present) – one review[26] detailed 2 broken needles and 4 infections in 17 500 reported blocks. Spray-as-you-go is particularly useful if cricothyroid puncture is not possible (local infection, abnormal anatomy, laryngeal pathology etc.); it is desirable to inspect endoscopically the anatomy before proceeding with intubation, or if it is unwise to anaesthetise the entire respiratory tract before intubation (aspiration risk).

Nebulization techniques are popular with some practitioners; the patient breathes an aerosol of lignocaine produced, usually, by placing 4% lignocaine in a gas driven nebulizer. However, better results are probably obtained with a 10% lignocaine solution that is not widely available. The process may take 20 minutes and nebulizers commonly used (e.g. for salbutamol) may not provide the correct particle size. Mean blood levels after nebulization with 10% lignocaine are not high.[27]

None of the techniques guarantee a lack of patient response, either to the procedure itself or topical anaesthetic administration. Topical anaesthesia to the nasal mucosa does not overcome the brisk sensation that occurs when a full-size tracheal tube is inserted fully through the nostril. Patients often wince at this point. Transtracheal injection and direct injection onto the cords of local anaesthetic promotes vigorous coughing. Nebulization may not produce adequate topical anaesthesia. A benzodiazepine produces amnesia and an opioid reduces the unpleasant sensation of tube passage. However, oversedation produces an uncooperative patient and is counterproductive. The benzodiazepines cause relaxation of the genioglossus muscle and promote central and obstructive hypopnoea, even in normal patients.[28] Administration of a benzodiazepine, and/or opioid can lead easily to a state indistinguishable from general anaesthesia.

DIFFICULT FIBREOPTIC INTUBATION

There are few formal studies on difficult fibreoptic intubation. One study[29] detailed the causes of difficulty found in a series of 423 consecutive nasotracheal intubations over a 4 year period. Virtually all patients were intubated awake after topical anaesthesia to the nose with cocaine and a translaryngeal injection of 3 ml of lignocaine 4%. The causes of difficulty described were: distortion of the airway due to septal deviation, oedema mass in the neck or oropharynx (16 patients), deviation of airway due to soft tissue contraction (4), decrease in space between the tip of the epiglottis and posterior pharyngeal wall (10), blood/secretions (8). Railroading the tracheal tube over a correctly placed fibrescope was not possible in three patients. A rare cause of difficult fibreoptic intubation, a cervical osteophyte, has been described recently. [30] The causes of difficult fibreoptic intubation and their possible solutions are given in Table 5.2.

Several techniques have been described that may aid fibreoptic intubation in difficult circumstances. An excellent article[31] describes the usefulness of transtracheal jet ventilation (TTJV) in difficult airway management and the equipment required. It is particularly useful in the cannot intubate/ cannot ventilate scenario which occurs with an incidence of 0.01–2.0 per 10 000 anaesthetics and is responsible for 1–28% of all deaths associated with anaesthesia. TTJV can provide a route for ventilation of a patient whilst elective fibreoptic intubation is undertaken. The technique is particularly useful in a patient in whom general anaesthesia is indicated for intubation, but in whom mask ventilation is likely to be difficult. The planned insertion of a catheter for transtracheal ventilation carries a low morbidity; this compares with the problems of emergency placement of such devices. Several reports describe the use of TTJV with fibreoptic intubation both with conventional rates of ventilation[32, 33] and with high frequency jet ventilation.[34] The practical steps are outlined in Table 5.3. It is particularly important to avoid vocal cord closure during TTJV; laryngospasm may lead to severe barotrauma.[35]

Retrograde cannulation by railroading a tracheal tube over a guide wire inserted percutaneously through the cricothyroid membrane into the oral cavity was described in 1960. The principles of combining this with fibreoptic intubation (Table 5.4) have been described in adults[36] and children.[37] A J-wire may be easier to find and grasp in the mouth. The cricotracheal route of retrograde cannulation may be safer.[38]

Failure to railroad the tube over the scope into the trachea is a common problem (Table 5.2). The bevel of the tube impinges on the larynx. An experimental tube with a tapered tip was virtually free of this problem.[39] A smaller tracheal tube inside the selected one[40, 41] or a commercially available blocker (Rusch UK) are helpful.

PAEDIATRICS

Fibreoptic intubation in babies and children poses several difficulties. The physical dimensions of the fibrescope limit the lower size of tracheal tube that can be used. The Olympus LF-2 has a nominal external diameter of 4 mm and will not accommodate a tube smaller than 4.5 mm. Even if a small diameter fibrescope is used, it is difficult to know the correct size of

Table 5.2 Common causes of difficult fibreoptic intubation and their solutions

Problem	Cause	Possible solutions
Misty view	Blood/secretions	Use an antisialogogue and demister Use suction catheter prior to endoscopy Blow 2–3 l/min oxygen down suction channel Use fibrescope before multiple blind intubation attempts Introduce fibrescope carefully under direct vision from the outset
Can't find larynx	Larynx displaced, floppy epiglottis, elevated posterior pharynx, redundant mucosal folds	Jaw thrust, tongue protrusion, use direct laryngoscope as well Sit patient up, or patient in lateral position Go round the edge of a large floppy epiglottis Retrograde wire technique
Can't identify larynx	Landmarks destroyed by tumour, oedema	Ask patient to vocalise or pant to identify vocal cord movement Look for bubbles indicating gas flow Inspect any 'hole' for visible tracheal rings
Can't railroad tube	Bevel of tube catching on larynx	Disimpact tracheal tube, rotate 90 degrees anticlockwise and reinsert Rotate tube continuously during advancement Use smaller tracheal tube inside selected one Use commercial tube blocker
Can't remove 'scope	Tube squashed/kinked	Do not try excessive force to extract scope – it will be damaged Use anterograde wire, remove scope and tube and reintubate over wire. Use armoured tracheal tube or size nostril with airway before endoscopy

Table 5.3 Steps for fibreoptic intubation with transtracheal ventilation

1 Topical anaesthesia of the trachea by transtracheal injection
2 Placement of transtracheal catheter in awake patient
3 Confirm ability to TTJV
4 Induction of anaesthesia with muscle relaxation
5 Confirm free egress of air through vocal cords to prevent barotrauma
6 Maintenance of IV anaesthesia, relaxation and ventilation (Anaesthetist 1)
7 Oral/nasal fibreoptic intubation (Anaesthetist 2)
8 Transtracheal catheter left in situ until after extubation

Table 5.4 Practical steps in a retrograde wire assisted fibreoptic intubation

1 Topical anaesthesia of mouth, glottis and trachea
2 Suitable cannula is inserted through the cricothyroid membrane
   aiming to pass cephalad in the midline between the cords
3 Free aspiration of air through the cannula to indicate placement in
   air passage rather than mucosa
4 Passage of long guide wire (preferably J-wire) through the cannula to
   pass into oral cavity
5 Guide wire passing from mouth is fed retrogradely through suction
   channel of fibrescope
6 Intubating fibrescope is introduced into mouth and passes along
   wire, guiding fibrescope to glottis
7 Cannula is withdrawn when viewed through the fibrescope
8 Wire is withdrawn into fibrescope when tip of 'scope is below the
   cords
9 'Scope passed to carina in normal fashion

tracheal tube to load on the scope. It is possible to reach the carina with the 'scope and to find that the selected tube is either too large to pass through the glottis or so large that there is no leak around the tube once it is placed in the trachea. Asleep intubation techniques are more suitable in this group of patients provided that mask inflation is possible when anaesthetised. There are various ways to circumvent these problems:

The Ultrathin Fibrescope. A fine 2 mm scope allows a smaller tube to be railroaded. These fine scopes do not possess a suction channel and have a much 'whippier' feel to them than the larger adult scopes. They are effective even in small neonates.[42]

Anterograde Seldinger Technique. This was first described by Stiles[43] in 1974 and is a useful technique. The fibrescope is positioned above the cords in the normal manner. A long guide wire passed through the suction channel is directed under vision into the distal trachea. The fibrescope is withdrawn, leaving the wire in situ. An appropriately sized tracheal tube is railroaded over the wire. The same technique can be used in adults although some difficulty can occur with railroading the tube over the wire. The wire can be stiffened appropriately by a ureteric catheter.[44]

ADULT AIRWAY MANAGEMENT (EXCLUDING DIFFICULT INTUBATION)

Fibreoptic skills are useful in a range of applications.[45]

Placement of double lumen tube (DLT)

The normal manner of insertion of a DLT is 'blind' placement in the trachea/bronchus and verification of correct positioning by chest movement/auscultation. This may be entirely inadequate. Alliaume and Colleagues placed DLTs in 24 patients by this blind technique and then evaluated the correct position of the tube by fibreoptic bronchoscopy.[46] Bronchoscopy led to the repositioning of 78% of left DLTs and 83% of right-sided tubes. Pooled results[47] from other studies confirm these findings, showing a repositioning rate of 58% (left) and 84% (right). Turning the patient laterally, or surgical manipulation, may also necessitate further fibreoptically-judged tube repositioning in 25% of patients. The criteria for correct placement are:

Via the tracheal lumen

This gives an unobstructed view of the tracheal carina and the non-intubated bronchus, and an endobronchial cuff positioned just below the carina, without herniation.

Via the bronchial lumen

This gives an absence of narrowing of the lumen by an overinflated bronchial cuff and an unobstructed view of the distal bronchial tree, including the upper lobe bronchus.

Correct placement of single lumen tracheal tube

Fibreoptic assessment of the correct placement of the tip of a tracheal tube in relation to the carina is accurate. [48] A 'routine' postintubation chest X-ray is not then necessary.

Correct placement of nasopharyngeal airway

Full insertion of standard nasopharyngeal tubes leads frequently to the tip lying distal to the epiglottis, or in the vallecula. Fibreoptic assessment of nasopharyngeal tube position in 120 patients found the incidence of these misplacements to be 60% and 13% respectively. [49]

Changing tracheal tubes

Changing tracheal tubes in ITU or the operating environment can be difficult. In ITU it is often necessary to discontinue ventilatory support for the minimum period. With the original tube still in situ and continuance of mechanical ventilation, the fibrescope with loaded replacement is threaded down the other nostril or mouth; the fibrescope tip is then positioned in the trachea outside the existing tube. The cuff of the original tube is deflated and the fibrescope tip passed to the carina. The original tube is removed and the new tube threaded over the inserted fibrescope.[50]

Trial of extubation

In some patients it is advantageous to insert the fibrescope through the tracheal tube prior to extubation. The tube and fibrescope are withdrawn together until both lie above the vocal cords. Assessment of airway oedema, narrowing, and vocal cord movement is possible. The fibrescope and tube are in position for immediate reinsertion should it be necessary.

Upper airway endoscopy

This may be useful in a wide range of conditions, including apparent upper airway obstruction resulting from infections, tumour, and abnormalities of vocal cord movement during or after thyroid surgery.[51] In respiratory burns, airway[52] endoscopy is particularly useful in determining the extent of involvement of the laryngeal area and in guiding placement of a tracheal tube before obstruction intervenes.

Lower airway endoscopy

Notably in patients with suspected tracheobronchial tears or respiratory distress due to tracheal narrowing. Loading of a tracheal tube prior to fibrescope insertion allows tracheal intubation to be undertaken under direct vision if required.

ACCIDENT AND EMERGENCY USE

The fibrescope has a small, but important, role in the management of patients attending accident and emergency departments. One study[53] reviewed all intubations undertaken in the emergency department over a 30 month period. Out of a total of 1862 intubations, 35 were undertaken fibreoptically. Four patients were trauma victims – two gunshot wounds to the neck, one orbital globe injury with clenched teeth and one flail chest with failed traditional intubation. The paper makes no convincing case that these patients were necessarily correctly managed by fibreoptic intubation. In particular, topical anaesthesia does not appear to have been used. The coughing produced by awake intubation attempts would have had adverse effects on the globe injury and could have initiated haemorrhage from the neck injury.

The use of fibreoptic intubation in *cervical spine trauma* is controversial.[54]

It is unfortunate that a major determinant of advised practice may be a consideration of medico-legal factors. An anaesthetist who has intubated such a patient awake and documented intact neurology postintubation cannot be blamed for neurological deterioration post-surgery. The real issue, however, is whether an awake fibreoptic-guided (rather than blind) intubation reduces the risk of intubation-related neurological deterioration when compared with intubation in the anaesthetised and paralysed patient. There is no clear consensus that this is true.

Awake intubation certainly seems to be safe, despite the theoretical problems of exacerbation of raised intracranial pressure, neck movement on coughing with topical anaesthetic administration and aspiration prior to intubation. A retrospective study[55] examined 454 patients with critical cervical cord/spine injury, of whom 165 underwent awake intubation within 2 months of injury. Neurological worsening following arrival in the hospital was seen in 2.4% of these patients, exactly the same rate as in the 289 patients who did not require intubation. Of the four patients who deteriorated in the intubation group, two deteriorated before intubation; both patients who deteriorated postintubation did so several hours later and had normal postintubation neurology.

If the patient is intubated under general anaesthesia, it is considered advisable for an assistant to provide manual in-line stabilization of the neck during intubation. This restriction of neck and head movement may make traditional laryngoscopy difficult. Simulation in normal patients of the desired intubation position for patients with cervical injuries, with cricoid pressure, showed an increased incidence of difficulty with intubation and the usefulness of a gum-elastic bougie in overcoming this problem.[56]

The management of the trauma patient with suspected neck injury has been reviewed[57, 58] and a critique of the ATLS recommendations in the context of British medical practice has been published.[59]

CARDIOVASCULAR CHANGES

Studies have demonstrated quite clearly that fibreoptic intubation alone (under general anaesthesia without topical anaesthesia) does not attenuate the cardiovascular changes when compared with direct laryngoscopy. Indeed, the changes may be more pronounced. Finfer and colleagues[60] found little difference between fibreoptic and traditional laryngoscopy, except in one subgroup in whom a more pronounced tachycardia was present 3–4 minutes after intubation fibreoptically. In both groups there were significant increases in heart rate and blood pressures following intubation. Smith[61] found greater heart rate and arterial pressure increases in the fibreoptic intubation group compared with traditional intubation. A subsequent study[62] from the same group showed that the means of oral fibreoptic intubation (tongue retraction versus Berman airway) did not influence the haemodynamic response.

The nature of the general anaesthetic technique probably does not influence the cardiovascular changes, except for the inclusion of opioids. A controlled study[63] compared total intravenous anaesthesia with enflurane anaesthesia and detected no difference between groups. The cardiovascular response to fibreoptic intubation under general anaesthesia can be attenuated by fentanyl 6 µg/kg[64] (the only dose studied) or alfentanil 10 µg/kg.[65] In the latter randomized, double-blind study, alfentanil in this dose abolished a rise in systolic blood pressure following intubation but only attenuated an increase in heart rate; mean heart rates of 90 beats/min (control) rose to 104 beats/min (alfentanil) and 117 beats/min (saline).

Awake intubation with full topical anaesthesia and sedation would appear to be the best option for cardiovascular stability. In one study[66] awake nasotracheal intubation was undertaken after instillation of cocaine (5%) to the nostrils, 4 ml lignocaine (4%) to the trachea via cricothyroid puncture and midazolam/fentanyl sedation. There were insignificant changes in systolic pressures and heart rate after intubation. Another study[67] looking at awake intubation detailed some increases in heart rate and systolic and diastolic blood pressures. Alfentanil (20 µg/kg) obtunded these changes but at the risk of respiratory depression.

RIGID INTUBATING FIBRESCOPES

Rigid fibrescopes combine a fibreoptic viewing bundle and eyepiece with an 'anatomically' curved, rigid blade. The scope is introduced into the mouth and the tip manipulated to lie just in front of the glottis utilizing the view though the viewing fibrebundle. The tracheal tube is then passed through the vocal cords, again under vision (unlike flexible fibreoptic intubation in which the tracheal tube is not seen to be passing through the cords). These scopes would appear to be particularly useful in patients with limited mouth opening, since a gap of about 12 mm only is required to introduce the scope into the mouth. They might be suitable for introduction into mainstream anaesthesia as a laryngoscope that is entirely suitable for routine cases, but is superior to direct laryngoscopy in many difficult cases. Flexible fibreoptic intubation has never made this jump from a specialist to a routine technique. Enthusiasts will take to rigid fibrescopes but it is not clear, presently, that their use will spread. In mannikins, rigid and flexible scopes require a similar amount of practice.[68]

The Bullard laryngoscope was designed to facilitate laryngoscopy and intubation in the difficult airway. Adult and paediatric versions have been evaluated. The tube requires a certain amount of manipulation to ensure that it passes between the cords; this manipulation is performed via intubating forceps, over a stylet or with a precurved tube. An early, small series[69] of 40 'normal' patients showed mean intubation times of 16 seconds. Three failures of intubation occurred in the first 10 patients. The authors had sufficient courage to use the scope in 10 rapid sequence inductions – fortunately without difficulty. The paediatric version was evaluated[70] in 93 children (mean age 2.1 years) of whom 29 were known, or expected, difficult laryngoscopy cases. Laryngoscopy was successful in 97% of patients in a mean time of 12.6 seconds (range 6–45 seconds). Only 15 of these patients required intubation and 14 were intubated without difficulty. The Bullard has also been evaluated in combination with jet ventilation of the trachea.[71]

The Upsherscope was designed by Dr M Upsher for routine intubation rather than specifically for difficult intubations. It is simpler to use than the Bullard because no formal tube manipulation is required. No studies have been published yet but several are in progress. In the author's experience, some patients in whom direct laryngoscopy is very difficult may be intubated easily with this scope.

The advantages of rigid scopes are that mouth opening and neck movement are much less important in determining successful intubation and the scope is robust, easy to clean and of a reasonably familiar shape for anaesthetists. The learning curve has yet to be determined for the Upsherscope, but appears steep for the Bullard. The introduction of the scope and vector of lift are different from that required with a direct laryngoscope. As with all fibreoptic instruments, blood and secretions make successful manipulations difficult and an antisialogogue is very useful.

DISINFECTION

Both rigid and flexible fibrescopes must be cleaned and disinfected after each patient.[72] The activated glutaraldehydes are the current disinfectants of choice for their spectrum of bactericidal, sporicidal and viricidal activity. However, exposure to the fluid or fumes may give rise to headache, nausea, eye irritation and occupational 'asthma'. The safe level according to Control of Substances Hazardous to Health UK regulations is 0.2 ppm. Peracetic acid is a new agent, yet to be formally introduced, that yields acetic acid and hydrogen peroxide. Disinfection can be accomplished in 10 minutes. The solution is only stable for 24 hours and is not compatible with brass and copper components of old style automated disinfection units.

KEY POINTS FOR CLINICAL PRACTICE

- It is essential to grasp the concept that the vector of view through the scope is not necessarily the vector of movement of the scope. If the tip is angulated, the view will appear to be straight ahead but it is actually to the side. If the scope is pushed in, the view will slide past rather than come closer. The scope is not an intelligent black snake that is dragged into the trachea by its flexible seeing head; it is pushed into position through the long axis of the scope.

- Start on patients by using either an asleep intubation technique that allows intubation and ventilation to occur simultaneously (with an independent anaesthetist looking after the patient) or on awake patients. The use of video facilities makes the learning/teaching process very much easier and you should try to use them whenever possible. You will learn more quickly and become less discouraged if a teacher can see the same view as you and direct your manipulations.
- Fibreoptic intubation consists of two separate skills – endoscopy to find/ traverse the larynx and railroading the tube over the inserted fibrescope. These skills do not have to be learnt at the same time; endoscopic competence is harder to acquire. It is possible, for teaching purposes, to endoscope a patient to find the larynx without committing yourself to full intubation.
- Secretion control is essential and patients should receive an antisialogogue. Thick secretions cannot be sucked up the suction channel of an intubating fibrescope because it is too narrow; use an ordinary suction catheter instead. Insufflation of 2–3 l/min oxygen down the suction channel helps to blow thin secretions away from the viewing lens. A proprietary demister is useful.
- Endoscopy begins at the lips or nares and should continue, ideally, under vision from there until the carina is reached; this minimizes fruitless and damaging mucosal contact. The vocal cords are reached usually within a distance of 15 cm from the external nares and it is useful to hold the scope at this distance from the tip to avoid oesophageal placement. In asleep techniques, jaw thrust by an assistant is essential to maintain the oro- or nasopharyngeal 'space'.
- After gaining some dexterity, practise fibreoptic intubation on routine patients who require intubation. It is quite in order to use the same anaesthetic technique as you would for traditional laryngoscopy because uncomplicated fibreoptic intubation takes 15–30 seconds only to complete. You do not need any special equipment or techniques once you have gained some familiarity with the device. There is no point in learning fibreoptic intubation and then never practising it.
- It is essential to be competent at awake intubations and to use awake techniques whenever the airway is, or is likely to be, difficult to manage. Sedation with benzodiazepines can easily turn an acceptable airway into an unstable one requiring emergency intervention. Do not sedate if the airway is compromised. Manouevres in difficult fibreoptic intubation such as sitting the patient up, asking the patient to pant or vocalize can only be undertaken in an awake patient. Awake techniques are easy to master and safe.
- Most difficult intubations in routine surgical patients can be mask ventilated easily. It doesn't matter whether these patients are intubated awake or asleep, although you must make a specific decision before using an asleep technique. However, difficult intubation inevitably overlaps with

difficult airway control and you need to be proficient in both areas. Remember the anterograde and retrograde wire techniques and the usefulness of establishing transtracheal ventilation electively in difficult cases. All the necessary equipment should be readily available in a dedicated trolley. Always confirm tracheal tube placement by capnography.

REFERENCES

1. Murphy P. A fiberoptic endoscope used for tracheal intubation. Anaesthesia 1967; 22: 489–491
2. Murphy P. Personal communication to Dr I Calder, 1990
3. Wood P R, Dresner M, Lawler P G P. Training in fibreoptic tracheal intubation in the North of England. Br J Anaesth 1992; 69: 202–203
4. Mason R A. Learning fibreoptic intubation: fundamental problems. Anaesthesia 1992; 47: 729–731
5. Vaughan R S. Training in fibreoptic laryngoscopy. Br J Anaesth 1991; 66: 538–540
6. Ovassapian A, Yelich S J, Dykes M H M, Golman M E. Learning fibreoptic intubation: use of simulators v. traditional teaching. Br J Anaesth 1988; 61: 217–220
7. Dykes M H M, Ovassapian A. Dissemination of fibreoptic airway endoscopy skills by means of a workshop utilizing models. Br J Anaesth 1989; 63: 595–597
8. Smith J E, Fenner S G, King M J. Teaching fibreoptic nasotracheal intubation with and without closed circuit television. Br J Anaesth 1993; 71: 206–211
9. Smith M, Calder I, Crockard A, et al. Oxygen saturation and cardiovascular changes during fibreoptic intubation under general anaesthesia. Anaesthesia 1992; 47: 158–161
10. Benumof J L. Use of the laryngeal mask airway to facilitate fiberscope-aided tracheal intubation. Anesth Analg 1992; 74: 313–314
11. Reynolds P I, O'Kelly S W. Fiberoptic intubation and the laryngeal mask airway. Anesthesiology 1993; 79: 1144
12. Hasham F, Kumar C M, Lawler P G P. The use of the laryngeal mask airway to assist fibreoptic orotracheal intubation. Anaesthesia 1991; 46: 891
13. Darling J R, Keohane M, Murray J M. A split laryngeal mask as an aid to training in fibreoptic tracheal intubation. Anaesthesia 1993; 48: 1079–1082
14. Alexander R, Moore C. The laryngeal mask airway and training in naso-tracheal intubation. Anaesthesia 1993; 48: 350–351
15. McCrirrick A, Pracilio J A. Awake intubation: a new technique. Anaesthesia 1991; 46: 661–663
16. Coe P A, King T A, Towey R M. Teaching guided fibreoptic nasotracheal intubation. An assessment of an anaesthetic technique to aid training. Anaesthesia 1988; 43: 410–413
17. Ralston S J, Charters P. Cuffed nasopharyngeal tube as 'dedicated airway' in difficult intubation. Anaesthesia 1994; 49: 133–136
18. Rooney R, Crummy E J, McShane A J. Bacteraemia following nasopharyngeal airway insertion. Anaesthesia 1992; 47: 1099
19. Nagaro T, Hamami G, Takasaki Y, Arai T. Ventilation via a mouth mask facilitates fiberoptic nasal tracheal intubation in anesthetized patients. Anesthesiology 1993; 78: 603–604
20. Williams L, Teague P D, Nagia A H. Foreign body from a Patil-Syracuse mask. Anesth Analg 1991; 73: 359–360
21. Yentis S M, Jankowski S, Gregory I C. Intermittent thiopentone for teaching fibreoptic nasotracheal intubation. Anaesthesia 1993; 48: 557–559
22. Schaefer H G, Marsch S C U, Keller H L, et al. Teaching fibreoptic intubation in anaesthetised patients. Anaesthesia 1994; 49: 331–334
23. Benumof J L. Management of the difficult adult airway with special emphasis on awake tracheal intubation. Anesthesiology 1991; 75: 1087–1110

24. Telford R J, Liban J B. Awake fibreoptic intubation. Br J Hosp Med 1991; 46:
    182–184
25. Sidhu V S, Whitehead E M, Ainsworth Q P et al. A technique of awake fibreoptic
    intubation: experience in patients with cervical spine disease. Anaesthesia 1993; 48:
    910–913
26. Gold M I, Buechel D R. Translaryngeal anesthesia. A review. Anesthesiology 1959;
    20: 181–185
27. Mostafa S M, Beese E. Plasma concentration of lignocaine after nebulization for
    awake fibreoptic intubation. Br J Anaesth 1993; 71: 759–760
28. Montravers P, Dureuil B, Desmonts J M. Effects of i.v. midazolam on upper airway
    resistance. Br J Anaesth 1992; 68: 27–31
29. Ovassapian A, Yelich S J, Dykes M H M, Brunner E E. Fiberoptic nasotracheal
    intubation-incidence and causes of failure. Anesth Analg 1983; 62: 692–695
30. Ranasinghe D N, Calder I. Large cervical osteophyte – another cause of difficult
    flexible fibreoptic intubation. Anaesthesia 1994; 49: 512–514
31. Benumof J L, Scheller M S. The importance of transtracheal jet ventilation in the
    management of the difficult airway. Anesthesiology 1989; 71: 769–778
32. Baraka A. Transtracheal jet ventilation during fiberoptic intubation under general
    anaesthesia. Anesth Analg 1986; 65: 1091–1092
33. Cooper D W, Long G T. Difficult fibreoptic intubation in an intellectually
    handicapped patient. Anaesth Intensive Care 1992; 20: 227–229
34. Boucek C D, Gunnerson H B, Tullock W C. Percutaneous transtracheal
    high-frequency jet ventilation as an aid to fiberoptic intubation. Anesthesiology
    1987; 67: 247–249
35. Schumacher P, Stotz G, Schneider M, Urwyler A. Laryngospasm during
    transtracheal high frequency jet ventilation. Anaesthesia 1992; 47: 855–856
36. Gupta B, McDonald J S, Brooks J H J, Mendenhall J. Oral fibreoptic intubation over
    a retrograde guidewire. Anesth Analg 1989; 68: 517–519
37. Audenaert S M, Montgomery C L, Stone B et al. Retrograde-assisted fiberoptic
    tracheal intuabtion in children with difficult airways. Anesth Analg 1991; 73:
    660–664
38. Shantha T R. Retrograde intubation using the subcricoid region. Br J Anaesth 1992;
    68: 109–112
39. Jones H E, Pearce A C, Moore P. Fibreoptic intubation. Influence of tracheal tube
    tip design. Anaesthesia 1993; 48: 672–674
40. Marsh N J. Easier fibreoptic intubations. Anesthesiology 1992; 76: 860–861
41. Oyston J, Hennessy M, Fisher J A. A double tube technique of adult fiberoptic
    assisted tracheal intubation. Anesthesiology 1992; 77: 1054–1056
42. Finer N N, Muzyka D. Flexible endoscopic intubation of the neonate. Pediatr
    Pulmonol 1992; 12: 48–51
43. Stiles C M. A flexible fiberoptic bronchoscope for endotracheal intubation of
    infants. Anesth Analg 1974; 53: 1017–1019
44. Telford R J, Searle J F, Boaden R W, Baier F. Use of a guide wire and a ureteral
    dilator as an aid to awake fibreoptic intubation. Anaesthesia 1994; 49: 691–693
45. Dellinger R P. Fiberoptic bronchoscopy in adult airway management. Crit Care Med
    1990; 18: 882–887
46. Alliaume B, Coddens J, Deloof T. Reliability of auscultation in positioning of
    double-lumen endobronchial tubes. Can J Anaesth 1992; 39: 687–690
47. Zbinden S. Fibreoptic bronchoscopy and double-lumen endobronchial tubes. Can J
    Anaesth 1993; 40: 681
48. Nielsen L H, Kristensen J, Knudsen F et al. Fibre-optic bronchoscopic evaluation of
    tracheal tube position. Eur J Anaesthesiol 1991; 8:277–279
49. Stoneham M D. The nasopharyngeal airway; assessment of position by fibreoptic
    laryngoscopy. Anaesthesia 1993; 48: 575–580
50. Smith J E, Fenner S G. Conversion of orotracheal to nasotracheal intubation with
    the aid of the fibreoptic laryngoscope. Anaesthesia 1993; 48: 1016
51. Akhtar T M. Laryngeal mask airway and visualisation of vocal cords during thyroid
    surgery. Can J Anaesth 1991; 38: 140
52. Masanes M-J, Legendre C, Lioret N et al. Fiberoptic bronchoscopy for the early

diagnosis of subglottal inhalation injury: comparative value in the assessment of prognosis. J Trauma 1994; 36: 59–67

53. Mlinek E J, Clinton J E, Plummer D, Ruiz E. Fiberoptic intubation in the emergency department. Ann Emerg Med 1990; 19: 359–362

54. Crosby E T. Tracheal intubation in the cervical spine-injured patient. Can J Anaesth 1992; 39: 105–107

55. Meschino A, Devitt J H, Koch J-P et al. The safety of awake tracheal intubation in cervical spine injury. Can J Anaesth 1992; 39: 114–117

56. Nolan J P, Wilson M E. Orotracheal intubation in patients with potential cervical spine injuries: an indication for the gum elastic bougie. Anaesthesia 1993; 48: 630–633

57. Hastings R H, Marks J D. Airway management for trauma patients with potential cervical spine injuries. Anesth Analg 1991; 73: 471–482

58. Criswell J C, Parr M J A, Nolan J P. Emergency airway management in patients with cervical spine injuries. Anaesthesia 1994; 49: 900–903

59. Wood P R, Lawler P G P. Managing the airway in cervical spine injury. A review of the advanced trauma life support protocol. Anaesthesia 1992; 47: 792–797

60. Finfer S R, MacKenzie S I P, Saddler J M, Watkins T G L. Cardiovascular responses to tracheal intubation: a comparison of direct laryngoscopy and fibreoptic intubation. Anaesth Intensive Care 1989; 17: 44–48

61. Smith J E. Heart rate and arterial pressure changes during fiberoptic tracheal intubation under general anaesthesia. Anaesthesia 1988; 43: 629-632

62. Smith J E, Mackenzie A A, Sanghera S S, Scott-Knight V C E. Comparison of two methods of fiberscope-guided tracheal intubation. Br J Anaesth 1991; 66: 546–550

63. Schaefer H-G, Marsch S C U, Strebel S P, Drewe J. Cardiovascular effects of fibreoptic oral intubation: a comparison of a total intravenous and a balanced volatile technique. Anaesthesia 1992; 47: 1034–1036

64. Smith J E, King M J, Yanny H F et al. Effect of fentanyl on the circulatory responses to orotracheal fibreoptic intubation. Anaesthesia 1992; 47: 20–23

65. Hartley M, Morris S, Vaughan R S. Teaching fibreoptic intubation: effect of alfentanil on the haemodynamic response. Anaesthesia 1994; 49: 335–337

66. Hawkyard J, Morrison A, Doyle L A et al. Attenuating the hypertensive response to laryngoscopy and endotracheal intubation using awake fibreoptic intubation. Acta Anaesthesiol Scand 1992; 36: 1–4

67. Randell T, Valli H, Lindgren L. Effects of alfentanil on the responses to awake fiberoptic nasotracheal intubation. Acta Anaesthesiol Scand 1990; 34: 59–62

68. Dyson A, Harris J, Bhatia K. Rapidity and accuracy of tracheal intubation in a mannequin; comparison of the fibreoptic with the Bullard laryngoscope. Br J Anaesth 1990; 65: 268–270

69. Saunders P R, Geisecke A H. Clinical assessment of the adult Bullard laryngoscope. Can J Anaesth 1989; 36: S118–S119

70. Borland L M, Casselbrant M. The Bullard laryngoscope; a new indirect oral laryngoscope (paediatric version). Anesth Analg 1990; 70: 105–108

71. Mendel P, Bristow A. Anaesthesia for procedures on the larynx and pharynx. The use of the Bullard laryngoscope in conjunction with high frequency jet ventilation. Anaesthesia 1993; 48: 263–265

72. Babb J R. Disinfection and sterilization of endoscopes. Curr Opinion Infect Disease 1993; 6: 532–537

6

R-R intervals and the depth of anaesthesia

C. J. D. Pomfrett

BACKGROUND

Depth of anaesthesia

One of the objectives of modern anaesthesia is to ensure that patients do not awaken inadvertently during surgery. This became a severe problem when competitive neuromuscular blockade was introduced in 1942, when, in conjunction with the use of opioid analgesics, most conventional signs of light anaesthesia, based on subjective estimates of pupillary diameter, movement and respiratory depression, were lost. Subjective measurements of anaesthetic depth taught routinely to medical students, such as Guedel's scale,[1] are therefore unreliable during modern anaesthetic practice. It has been suggested that there are four levels of awareness in patients under general anaesthesia:[2] conscious awareness with recall; conscious awareness without recall; subconscious awareness with recall; no awareness. Awareness can only occur if the sensory centres of the brain are functioning, and recall similarly requires that memory processes are still functioning during anaesthesia. Some contemporary estimates of the incidence of awareness during anaesthesia are listed in Table 6.1.

The lowest estimate of awareness, based on structured interviews, is still unacceptably high, at around 0.2%.[3] In order to reduce the incidence of awareness, there have been considerable efforts directed at the development of an objective monitor of anaesthetic depth.[4] No single method of measuring the depth of anaesthesia has been adopted, leaving the unfortunate situation that, despite the development of advanced anaesthetic agents allowing rapid recovery, the anaesthetist is still unable to measure the depth

Table 6.1 Incidence of awareness. Summary of incidence of awareness with recall and dreaming in studies using a structured interview[3]

Author	Date	Awareness (%)	Dreaming (%)	Sample Size
Hutchinson	1960	1.2	3	656
Harris	1971	1.6	26	120
McKenna	1973	1.5	–	200
Wilson	1975	0.8	7.7	490
Liu et al	1990	0.2	0.9	1000

of anaesthesia in order to prevent inadvertent awakening during anaesthesia. It has been suggested that anaesthesia is a continuum,[5] but there is no absolute unit of anaesthetic depth with which to mark progress along the continuum, making cross-patient comparisons of absolute depth impossible. The main reason is that attempts to quantify the depth of anaesthesia have been in the form of scales of visible effects of anaesthetic agents on a patient. If these visible effects, subjectively measured by an observer, are masked by another drug or an unrelated condition of the patient, the measurement of anaesthetic depth is invalidated. Putative tests of anaesthetic depth have to be tested against some 'gold standard' of anaesthetic depth. The most likely candidate is positron emission tomography (PET) where brain metabolism is accurately assessed during anaesthesia by measuring the regional uptake of radiolabelled sugars.[6] Unfortunately, PET scanners are expensive to run, require the availability of a nearby cyclotron to prepare short half-life isotopes and are not conveniently placed in operating theatres.

There has been considerable interest in the development of objective, electrophysiological measurements of anaesthetic depth. All of these measurements have focussed on elucidating brain function in a non-invasive manner. Several criteria have to be applied to any putative depth of anaesthesia monitor, the most important to an anaesthetist being ease of use and reliability. A monitor that is difficult to use or takes an inordinate time to set up for each patient will only be used rarely, and an unreliable monitor will not meet commercial or government requirements for certification.

The electroencephalogram (EEG) shows activity in the upper few millimetres of the cerebral cortex, for a region in the vicinity of the scalp recording electrodes, and will reflect the functional state of these areas of the brain. However, PET studies of brain metabolism have confirmed that the effects of contemporary anaesthetics are not evenly distributed throughout the brain.[6] It is, therefore, possible for specific regions of the brain to be functional during deep anaesthesia. This has been shown to be the case by the use of evoked potentials, where EEG responses to repetitive sensory stimuli are time-locked to the stimulus and averaged. It has been shown that the auditory pathway exhibits a dose-related reduction in activity with increasing levels of anaesthesia.[7] However, there are a number of drawbacks preventing the routine use of EEG-based monitoring techniques in the operating theatre. EEG recordings are distorted when made with ECG electrodes, and silver/silver chloride cup electrodes should be applied to skin which has been abraded in order to ensure a low impedance between the electrode and the skin, enhancing the amplitude of the EEG. This preparation takes time, patience and expertise, which is often not available in the anaesthetic room. The EEG electrodes are also prone to accidental loosening, which may increase skin impedance and give a false impression of the presence of a signal when it is actually electrical noise. Electrocautery (diathermy) is an example of an electronic countermeasure deployed by surgeons that prevents accurate EEG recordings, since the interference from electrocautery is many times greater than the amplitude of the EEG. Frequent electrocautery renders EEG recordings unusable. Even without such artefacts, the EEG has been shown to be affected by drugs in common use during anaesthesia, atropine causing significant increases in θ activity and decreases in β activity when measured in unanaesthetised volunteers.[8] The same study also discussed reductions in the amplitude and latency of the P300 cognitive potential by hyoscine, an atropine-like drug. In addition, it has been suggested that changes in blood sugar levels affect the evoked potential,[9] as will a break in the sensory pathway contributing to the AEP, e.g. deafness will prevent the determination of an auditory evoked potential.

The minimum alveolar concentration (MAC) of an anaesthetic agent predicts the amount of anaesthetic required to prevent movement to a noxious stimulus in 50% of patients. It has been shown that MAC can be measured in decerebrate rats, and, in addition, the presence of a cerebral cortex did not affect the level of MAC.[10] This gave an explanation as to why direct correlates of MAC could not be determined using the EEG alone.[11] This finding is particularly interesting when the action of some anaesthetic agents has been suggested to involve the brainstem,[12] the consequence being that inhibition in the brainstem is activated by the anaesthetic, and that the inhibition then reduces cerebral activity. If this is indeed the case, any monitor of cerebral activity will, at best, warn of the potential for awareness during anaesthesia at that moment, but will not predict it in advance if the underlying control of anaesthesia originates in the brainstem. In this circumstance the anaesthetist needs to open a window onto the regions of the brainstem affected by anaesthesia and responsible for activation of the cerebral cortex, which will mirror MAC on a physiological level and give the potential for predicting impending light anaesthesia. Such a monitor should allow MAC equivalent cross-agent comparisons of equipotency, and should, therefore, be of use for any of the different types of anaesthetic that could be given a conventional MAC or equivalent intravenous value.

Heart rate variability (HRV)

Heart rate changes during anaesthesia as a result of shifting balance between sympathetic excitation and parasympathetic inhibition of the heart. It is well established that tachycardia due to increasing sympathetic tone may be indicative of lightening anaesthesia. However, the mean heart rate cannot be used as a sole indicator of anaesthetic depth. This is because many of the drugs given during anaesthesia, including analgesics, alter the heart rate. For example, atropine reduces parasympathetic tone and is used to counteract bradycardia induced by excessive parasympathetic tone, so any method of determining the depth of anaesthesia by measuring the mean heart rate alone would fail during the use of atropine.

Studies on heart rate variability typically consider not the mean heart rate, but the instantaneous heart rate from beat to beat. If a tachygram of instantaneous heart rate against time is plotted, it is apparent that frequent small changes in the heart rate are present. This behaviour is typical of biological control loops, and has characteristics of a chaotic system. Small changes in instantaneous heart rate are invisible on a modern, rolling ECG monitor, but triggering an oscilloscope-type display with a fixed time base against one R-wave readily, but subjectively, shows HRV as a shifting second QRS complex. The level of HRV tends to decrease with increasing respiratory rate, the peak level of HRV being noted at around 5 breaths per minute.[13] Increased sympathetic tone and decreased parasympathetic tone with age results in an age-related reduction in the level of HRV, and this may be a consequence of decreased baroreceptor sensitivity due to age-related thickening of artery walls. No sex-related differences in the level of HRV have been reported.

Widespread interest in using HRV as an index of anaesthetic depth began in 1985, when an off-line study led to the suggestion that on-line monitoring of respiratory sinus arrhythmia (RSA), the high frequency respiratory component of HRV, could be used as an index of the level of anaesthesia.[14] The potential commercial significance of this observation is reflected in the filing of at least four patents based on methods of monitoring heart rate variability, three of which refer directly to the measurement of anaesthetic depth.[15-18]

One of the main areas of non-anaesthetic related research into HRV has been its use as a screen for autonomic neuropathy, especially during diabetes. The level of HRV falls rapidly during diabetes, due to a reduction in parasympathetic tone.[13] Significant reductions in RSA have been observed within 1 to 2 years after the diagnosis of diabetes mellitus.[19] This reduction in RSA was not a result of volume depletion. As the condition progresses, sympathetic tone then also falls, until on eventual denervation of the heart, there is no HRV. The pathogenesis of this neuropathy in neurones includes: microvascular lesions in autonomic ganglia and small nerves; metabolic disruption of neurones, including a build up of sorbitol and fructose as a result of exposure to high levels of glucose; lipid abnormalities due to a lack of insulin.[20] Morphological changes in these neurones include demyelination, degeneration of nerve roots and ganglia, and the presence of large vacuoles in cell bodies. Alcohol abuse and uraemia can also lead to reductions in HRV.[13]

Anaesthesia may potentially alter the level of HRV for a number of reasons:[21] the balance between sympathetic and parasympathetic tone may be altered; baroreceptor sensitivity may be altered; the anaesthetics may have depressant effects on reflex pathways at peripheral and ganglionic sites; central sites (e.g. brainstem) may be affected by the anaesthetic leading to altered integration of reflex activity. In order to identify these effects, it has been necessary to fully characterize the components of HRV. Objective methods used to accurately characterize the level of HRV and its components are discussed below.

Baroreceptor reflex

The baroreceptor reflex connects blood pressure sensors at the carotid sinus with the medulla of the brainstem.[22] Increased blood pressure at the carotid sinus causes increased vagal parasympathetic outflow and decreased sympathetic outflow slowing the heart and reducing blood pressure. The brainstem region for this activity is the solitary nucleus, effecting vagal activity via interneurones innervating the vagal motor nucleus. In addition, peripheral resistance is also controlled from the solitary nucleus via interneurones to the rostral ventrolateral medulla, from whence reticulospinal tract interneurones stimulate sympathetic ganglia, which affect arterioles and decrease peripheral resistance, therefore reducing blood pressure. The baroreceptor reflex is slow compared with other components of heart rate variability, and comprises a frequency band ranging from 0.05 to 0.15 Hz. Slower frequencies (<0.03 Hz) are rejected from most studies on HRV.[21] It has been suggested that thermoregulation and the renin-angiotensin system cause the very low frequency components of HRV.

Respiratory sinus arrhythmia

In the supine human, respiratory sinus arrhythmia (RSA) is characterized by an increase in instantaneous heart rate during inspiration and a decrease during expiration. This is demonstrated in Figure 6.1.

Stretch receptors in the lungs, chest wall and heart are activated during inspiration, and cause an increase in afferent activity to the medulla.[13] Neurones in the solitary nucleus inhibit tonically active vagal outflow to the heart, and the heart rate increases. There is also a minor increase in sympathetic outflow, which tends to increase the heart rate. RSA is typically measured as a high frequency component of heart rate variability, above 0.15 Hz.[21]

METHODS OF EXAMINING HEART RATE VARIABILITY

Several different approaches have evolved to study heart rate variability. Figure 6.2 demonstrates several of the techniques used to generate data from one patient undergoing anaesthesia with isoflurane.

The ideal method of quantifying heart rate variability will eliminate the need for time-consuming visual review of raw data, distinguish changes in R-R intervals due to pathological arrhythmia from changes due to autonomic balance, and provide a reliable real-time display that may be used by the average anaesthetist.

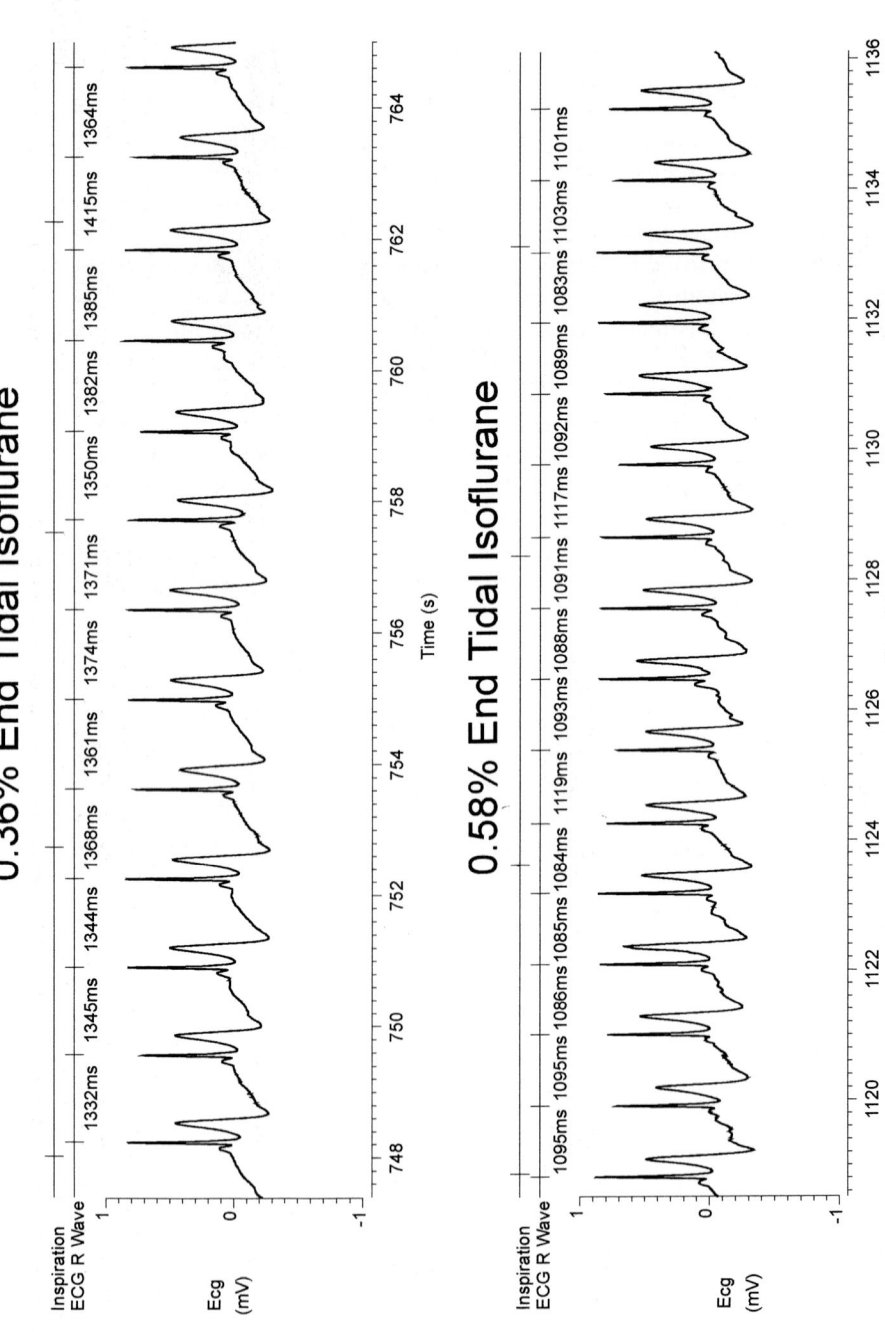

Figure 6.1 Examples of ECG traces (lead III) demonstrating heart rate variability (HRV) for the same patient (63 years old, ASA II) during anaesthesia at 0.36% and 0.58% end-tidal isoflurane. The ECG R-wave detection was performed on-line using template matching pattern recognition software. Note that HRV is difficult to recognize from the ECG waveforms alone.

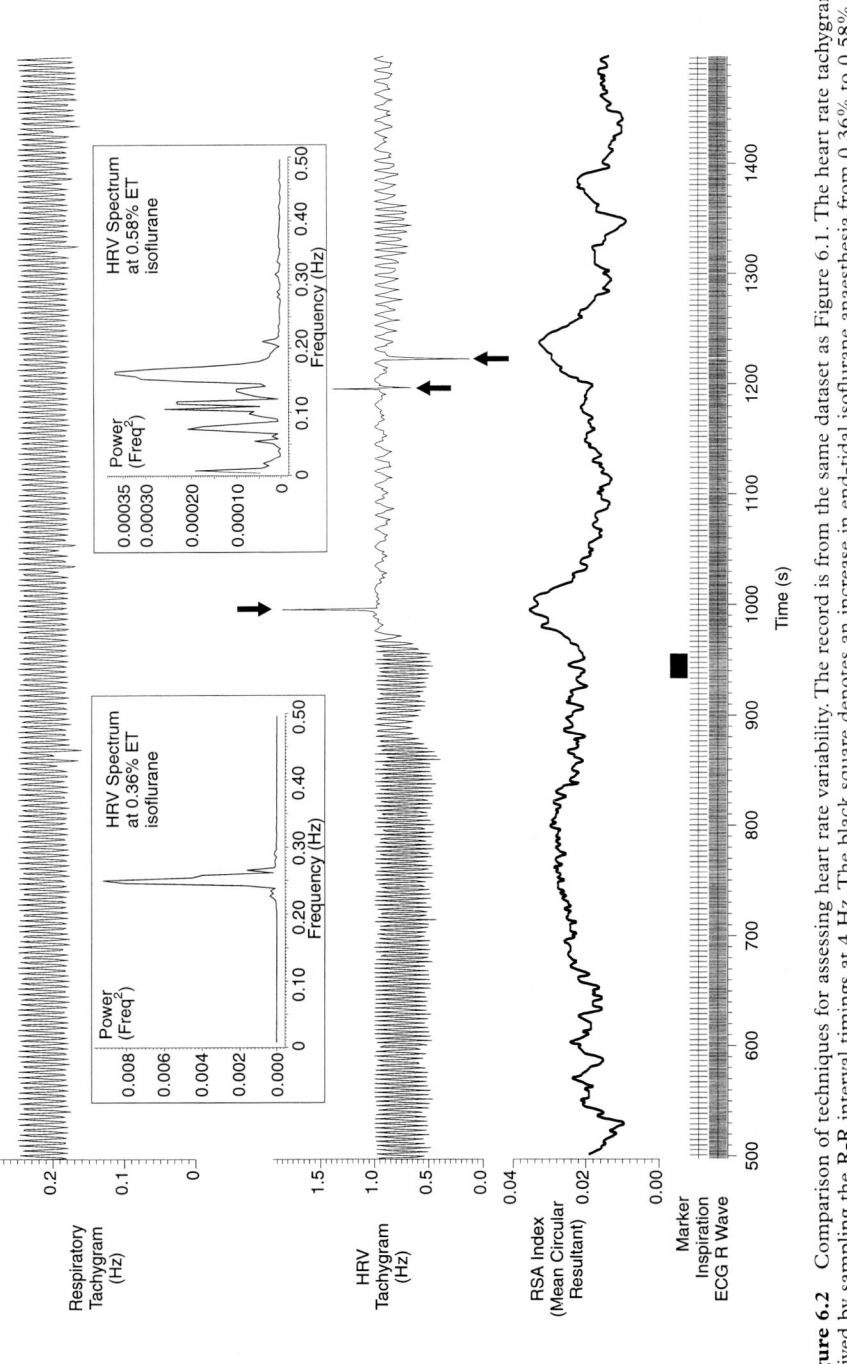

Figure 6.2 Comparison of techniques for assessing heart rate variability. The record is from the same dataset as Figure 6.1. The heart rate tachygram is derived by sampling the R-R interval timings at 4 Hz. The black square denotes an increase in end-tidal isoflurane anaesthesia from 0.36% to 0.58%. Respiratory sinus arrhythmia (RSA) decreased, and the inset power spectral analyses demonstrate that power shifted from respiratory frequencies (~0.25Hz) to attenuated, lower frequencies after anaesthesia increased. The mean circular resultant (shown as a moving average of 20 points) also showed a decrease in mean level from 0.0197 to 0.0171. Note that the mean circular resultant is calculated in real-time every 6 seconds, whereas the FFT-based spectral analysis requires a sampling epoch of 512 seconds. Arrows denote the presence of ectopic beats that must be rejected from the analysis.

Linear analysis

The simplest methods of analysing heart rate variability include simple statistics on the beat-to-beat intervals. The standard deviation from the mean of the R-R interval increases with an increase in heart rate variability.[23] However, this estimate does not discriminate between different components of heart rate variability. In addition, the standard deviation from the mean heart rate will become smaller as heart rate increases simply because a greater number of heart beats are included in the analysis.[13]

The Valsalva manoeuvre is where the baroreceptor response to forced breathing against resistance is measured.[20] Tachycardia and peripheral vasoconstriction are observed during the forced breathing, and after release there is an overshoot rise in blood pressure and bradycardia. Commonly, the ratio of longest R-R interval after the interval is measured against the shortest R-R interval during the manoeuvre. A low ratio suggests that there was no HRV. The Valsalva manoeuvre has limited use during anaesthesia, but may be used before anaesthesia begins to screen for patients with no HRV. However, this sort of measurement is very susceptible to contamination by ectopic beats.

Spectral analysis

A tachygram of the instantaneous heart rate is comprised of many component frequencies. Spectral analysis of the waveform identifies the components of the tachygram. There are typically three frequency bands, representing very low frequency circadian effects, medium frequency baroreceptor activity, and high frequency RSA.[21] The Fast Fourier Transform (FFT) is frequently used as a tool to extract the spectral components.[24] There are a number of conditions that the data must meet in order to use the FFT: data must be stationary, i.e. the spectral components of the data should not change during a sampling epoch or interval; the data should be sampled at frequencies that are at least double the highest frequency of interest; and the data should be low pass filtered at half the sampling frequency (the Nyquist frequency). A detailed comparison of several time and frequency domain techniques for measuring HRV has been conducted.[25] The authors suggested that all tested linear and spectral techniques gave comparable estimates of vagal tone by observing the high frequency, respiratory (RSA) component. However, frequency domain analysis of low frequencies did not correlate with vagal tone and were related to the control of blood pressure (Meyer waves).

Moving polynomial

In order to remove the requirement of stationary data, a prerequisite of spectral techniques, a method was developed and patented that extracted RSA from a moving polynomial of R-R data.[15] The technique functions in real-time, and has formed the basis for a commercial monitor of vagal tone (Vagal Tone Monitor, Delta-Biometrics Inc., Bethseda, Md., USA).

Circular analysis

Circular analysis is a different approach to the analysis of HRV.[19] It was first used to observe the extent of loss of RSA, and hence vagal tone, during the onset of autonomic neuropathy in diabetics. Circular analysis was used as a tool to dissect RSA from HRV and other arrhythmias. Table 6.2 shows the relative contribution of potential artefacts to the measurement of RSA.[13]

Circular analysis exploits the link between RSA and respiration. The onset of each inspiration is considered as the start of a circle, and the timings of ECG R-waves are plotted as vectors around the circle. The magnitude of each R-wave vector was one, and its angle depended on the relative position of the R-wave within the breath, e.g. the angle of an R-wave half way through breath would be 180°. The end of the circle is the start of the next inspiration. Weinberg and Pfeifer chose to fix the duration of breathing by asking their subjects to breathe at a frequency dictated by an oscilloscope.[19] They proposed that, in subjects where the breathing period could not be fixed, the circle's circumference could be normalized. This normalization is of obvious application with spontaneously breathing but anaesthetised patients.

RSA is apparent as an increase in clustering of R-wave timings into one point of the circle. RSA in the supine subject will lead to clustering during inspiration, i.e. within the first 180° of the circle. However, the clustering may occur randomly in a single breath due to non-respiratory arrhythmias,

Table 6.2 Comparison of methods of measuring respiratory sinus arrhythmia.[13] The ideal method would answer no to all questions

Method	Linked to intrinsic heart rate?	Affected by ectopic beats?	Affected by changes in average heart rate during the study?
Standard deviation from the mean R-R interval	Yes	Yes	Yes
Mean circular resultant (circular statistics)	No	Minimally	No
Maximum-minimum R-R interval	Yes	Yes	Slightly
Expired: Inspiratory ratio	Minimally	Yes	No
Holter monitoring	Yes	Yes	Yes
FFT spectral analysis	Yes*	Yes	Yes**

* the effects of intrinsic heart rate can be removed from the spectral analysis off-line.
** FFT-based spectral analysis requires that data is stationary.

so it was usual to average several, successive breaths. Derivation of the mean circular resultant allows RSA to be 'dissected' out from HRV using a numerically simple algorithm that is readily incorporated into an on-line monitoring system. Application of relevant statistics such as Rayleigh's test allows the anaesthetist to validate RSA data on-line, permitting the instant, automated rejection of bad data. This is a significant advance on FFT-based spectral techniques, where any contamination within a sampling epoch invalidates the analysis, which may typically be some 8 minutes of data. However, the mean circular resultant has the disadvantage that it does not reflect activity from the baroreceptor reflex that is revealed by spectral analysis.

RESULTS OF EXAMINING HEART RATE VARIABILITY

Table 6.3 shows the effects of some of the drugs used to determine the mechanisms underlying heart rate variability. Several studies have used these drugs during anaesthesia to eliminate parasympathetic and/or sympathetic components from the effects of anaesthesia alone. Beta-adrenergic block-ade leads to a small decrease in HRV.[13] Isoprenaline acts on the sympa-thetic receptors at the heart, increases heart rate and reduces HRV.

Baroreceptor reflex

The α-adrenergic agonist phenylephrine increases blood pressure and leads to a baroreceptor-mediated slowing of the heart rate. HRV tends to in-crease, and is parasympathetically mediated since atropine abolishes the increase in HRV. The α-adrenergic blocker phenylamine leads to the op-posite effect, decreasing blood pressure and leading to a baroreceptor-mediated increase in heart rate. HRV tends to decrease, and the decrease can be blocked by using propranolol to mask the change in the sympa-thetic nervous system.

The effect of isoflurane on the baroreceptor reflex has been studied in some detail.[26] This study examined the effects of isoflurane at 1.0 and 1.5

Table 6.3 Effects of drugs used to understand heart rate variability[13]

Drug	General effects	Effect on heart rate	Effect on HRV
Atropine	Decreases parasympathetic tone	Increases	Decreases
Isoprenaline Infusion	Increases cardiac sympathetic tone	Increases	Decreases
Propanolol Infusion	Decreases cardiac sympathetic tone	Decreases	Decreases
Phenylephrine Infusion	Increases blood pressure	Decreases	Increases
Phenylamine Infusion	Decreases blood pressure	Increases	Decreases

MAC on the baroreceptor reflex. The method used was to perform least squares regression analysis on the linear region of the sigmoidal relation between blood pressure and R-R interval. Three methods were used to induce the baroreceptor reflex: neck suction; pressor tests, where phenylephrine was infused; depressor tests, where sodium nitroprusside was infused. A progressive reduction in the baroreceptor reflex was observed as anaesthesia was increased from 1.0 to 1.5 MAC, which was less marked than the reduction observed during halothane and enflurane anaesthesia. The low frequency (baroreceptor) region of HRV was observed to reduce significantly in another study at induction with propofol and thiopentone, but no significant reduction was observed for etomidate.[27]

Respiratory sinus arrhythmia

Spectral analysis of the high frequency component of RSA has shown that it decreases significantly at induction with propofol and thiopentone, but no significant change was observed at induction with etomidate.[27] Spectral analysis revealed reduced high frequency components during thiopentone/N_2O anaesthesia, increased high frequency components during sufentanil anaesthesia and no change in parasympathetic/sympathetic balance during etomidate/N_2O anaesthesia.[21] The author suggested that either etomidate does not cause a reduction in HRV or etomidate may result in transient cortical stimulation that offsets depressant effects of a lack of consciousness on HRV.

Linear, dose-related reductions in the level of RSA have been observed using spectral analysis of HRV with isoflurane anaesthesia at 1.0, 1.5, and 2.0 MAC isoflurane in patients subjected to controlled ventilation.[28] The authors noted that the changes in HRV could be detected by visual inspection of the ECG. An on-line method has been developed for the determination of HRV spectra, giving a 3D compressed spectral array.[29] High frequency components of HRV, attributed with HRV, were observed to decline with deepening anaesthesia. However, any spectral technique needs a sampling epoch, in this case 256 seconds. Even if a sliding epoch is used, the relative contribution of a rapid, but transient, increase in RSA will not make a significant change immediately in the compressed spectral array.

Determination of RSA during anaesthesia has been performed in two studies using the moving polynomial technique.[15] In the first study, on ten patients anaesthetised with isoflurane/N_2O, RSA was depressed by 71% during maintenance of anaesthesia.[14] During recovery, vagal tone increased and approached the level seen at pre-induction of anaesthesia. In the second study, during enflurane/N_2O anaesthesia, vagal tone was reduced by 90% from baseline values.[30]

The mean circular resultant has been used in a number of studies on patients undergoing routine anaesthesia. This technique has the advantage of real time, on-line display to the anaesthetist, obtained from 30 second epochs. Ten patients (ASA I-II, gynaecological surgery) were studied during stepped propofol infusion.[31] Figure 6.3 shows a chart of grouped data from these patients, obtained during a two minute epoch after the change in anaesthetic concentration. Induction of anaesthesia was accompanied with a transient increase in the level of RSA, which then fell from baseline values in a dose-related manner. The median frequency of the EEG, another potential method of measuring the depth of anaesthesia, was also measured in these patients. The median frequency did not change in a consistent manner within the 2 minute sampling epochs. Recovery from anaesthesia was associated with a transient increase in the level of RSA to greater than baseline levels, which then returned to baseline levels after recovery. This transient increase makes the mean circular resultant a potential monitor of awakening from anaesthesia, in addition to staging anaesthetic depth. Figure 6.3 demonstrates the increase in RSA observed when propofol infusion syringe pump was recharged, but not switched back on. Within 2 minutes, the level of RSA rose significantly. Since this was a real-time display, the anaesthetist was alerted to the rise in vagal tone. The anaesthetic equipment was then checked, and the pump was switched back on. The patient was subject to competitive neuromuscular blockade and controlled ventilation, so that other signs of wakening were masked. It is possible that this is the first case when RSA has been used to avoid an incident of awareness under anaesthesia. The vagal tone took around 9 minutes to return back to predicted levels, based on the previous 15 minutes of anaesthesia. This suggested that there was a hysteresis in the response, with more rapid rises in vagal tone being observed during recovery from propofol anaesthesia. This is an opposite hysteresis to that seen with the EEG, which rapidly responds to deepening levels of anaesthesia but which responds more slowly to recovery. It was observed that the presence of surgical stimulation enhanced the level of vagal tone. This has also been reported in two other studies.[32,33] Figure 6.4 shows the effect of changing the level of isoflurane/N_2O anaesthesia.[34] The level of RSA fell in a dose dependent manner with increasing levels of anaesthesia, as did the median frequency of the EEG. However, surgical stimulation caused the level of RSA to rise, whereas the median frequency of the EEG was unaffected by surgical stimulation. This supports the concept that RSA is a more able indicator of MAC than the EEG.

Patients undergoing Caesarean section are particularly prone to suffering from awareness during surgery owing to the deliberately light anaesthesia given to protect the baby. One study using the mean circular resultant, demonstrated that the light anaesthesia and surgical stimulation associated with Caesarean section were reflected in high levels of vagal tone.[35]

CONCLUSION

Considerable efforts are being directed towards the development of closed-loop systems for the control of anaesthesia. It is likely that, in order to

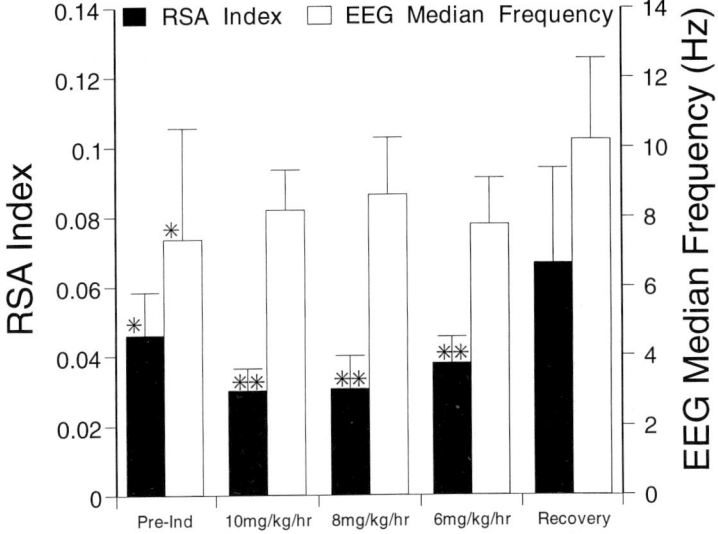

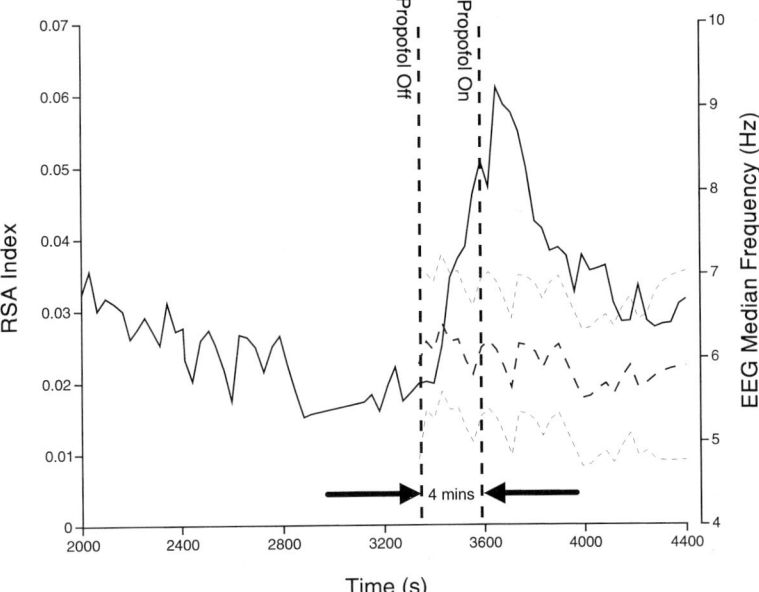

Figure 6.3   Upper. Comparison between two putative measurements of anaesthetic depth during propofol anaesthesia. Ten patients were anaesthetised with continuous infusions of propofol and the grouped respiratory sinus arrhythmia (RSA, mean circular resultant method) and EEG (median frequency) data were derived. Stars denote significant differences from recovery (*=P<0.05, **=P<0.01). (Graph redrawn from original data presented first in reference 31.) **Lower.** Time course of RSA (mean circular resultant method) during accidental interruption of propofol infusion. Dotted lines denote predicted behaviour of RSA ±99% confidence limits. RSA increased significantly above the predicted values 2 minutes after interruption of infusion. (Graph redrawn from original data presented first in reference 31.)

satisfy the criteria of safety criticality, several techniques for measuring the depth of anaesthesia will be combined. It is possible that measurement of parasympathetic tone will be partnered with measurements of cerebral activity such as the EEG, so that in the event that one measurement is unreliable, e.g. the patient has an abnormal EEG or autonomic neuropathy, the other technique will still be available.

The availability of a readily-determined index of activity in the brainstem will give a physiological analogue to MAC, and will probably permit the quantification of anaesthetic depth. An absolute, standardized physiological scale to describe the continuum that is anaesthetic depth is necessary to facilitate the adoption of monitoring to prevent awareness of patients during anaesthesia. In order to quantify the depth of anaesthesia, an absolute scale of cerebral and brainstem activity needs to be adopted. The most encouraging method of determining brain activity to date is to measure the uptake of radiolabelled sugars using PET scanning. PET scans are able to derive an absolute estimate of anaesthetic efficacy, but long scan times, invasive use of radioactive isotopes, and cost mean that PET will not be routinely used in the operating theatre based on current technology. Measurement of RSA using a scale of anaesthetic depth originally calibrated using PET may be part of the cost-effective alternative for routine determination of an aesthetic depth in the operating theatre of the future.

KEY POINTS FOR CLINICAL PRACTICE

- Sudden, unexplained changes in heart rate variability (HRV) during anaesthesia should not be ignored, since they may indicate a change in autonomic balance indicative of light anaesthesia.
- HRV can be subjectively observed by the use of an ECG monitor with a fixed, not rolling, timebase.
- Dedicated facilities allowing the measurement of HRV are desirable, value added options, available with some ECG monitoring systems.
- HRV includes respiratory sinus arrhythmia (RSA), bradycardia, tachycardia and other arrhythmias. In order to isolate vagal tone, a dedicated monitor of RSA has to be applied to the HRV data.
- HRV will be unreliable in patients with autonomic neuropathy or after heart transplantation. Alcoholism may lead to a loss of HRV, as may uraemia.
- Fast Fourier Transform (FFT) spectral techniques require stationary data where mean heart rate is not varying during a sampling epoch or interval.
- Some methods of determining RSA are more resilient to artefacts such as arrhythmias and ectopic beats than others, e.g. the mean circular resultant is more robust than using the standard deviation from the mean R-R interval.

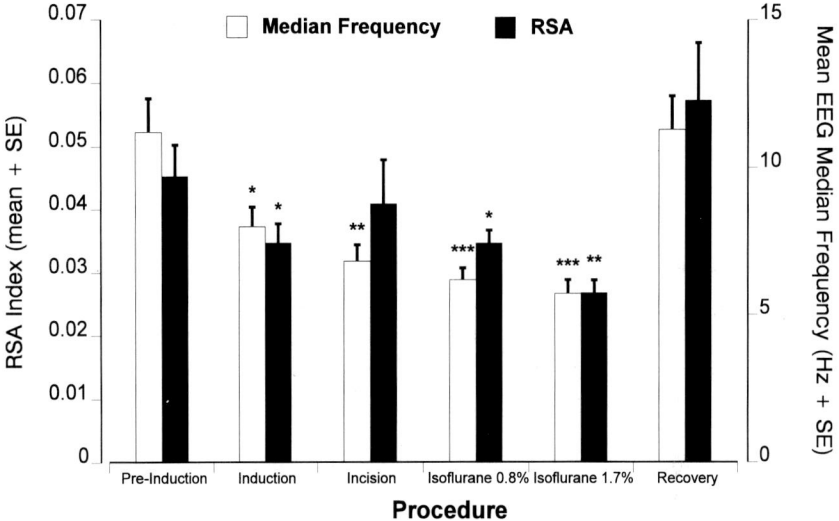

Figure 6.4 Comparison between two putative measurements of anaesthetic depth during isoflurane anaesthesia. Ten patients were anaesthetised with propofol and anaesthesia was maintained with 0.8% (0.65 MAC) and 1.7% (1.2 MAC) isoflurane steps. The grouped RSA (mean circular resultant) and EEG median frequencies were obtained. Stars denote significant differences from recovery (*=P<0.05, **=P<0.01, ***=P<0.001). (Graph redrawn from original data presented first in reference 34.)

REFERENCES

1. Guedel A. Third-stage ether anaesthesia: a subclassification regarding the significance of the position and movements of the eyeball. Am J Surg, Quarterly Supplement in Anaesthesia 1920; 34: 53–57
2. Jones J G. Depth of Anaesthesia. In: Ballière's Clinical Anaesthesiology, editorial. Ballie`re Tindall, London, 1989; 3(3): editorial
3. Liu, W H D, Thorp T A S, Graham S G, Aitkenhead A R. Incidence of awareness with recall during general anaesthesia. Anaesthesia 1991; 46: 435–437
4. Pomfrett C J D. Measurement of anaesthetic depth. Aether 1994; 1: 18–22
5. White D C. Anaesthesia: a privation of the senses. An historical introduction and some definitions. In: Rosen M, Lunn J N (eds) Conscious Awareness and Pain in General Anaesthesia. Butterworth, London, 1987
6. Alkire M T, Barker S J, Haier R J et al. A positron emission tomography study of cerebral metabolism in a volunteer during propofol anesthesia. Anesth Analg 1994; 78: S5
7. Thornton C, Newton D E F. The auditory evoked response: a measure of depth of anaesthesia. Ballière's Clinical Anaesthesiology 1989; 3(3): 559–585
8. Pickworth W B, Herning R I, Koeppl B, Henningfield J E. Dose-dependent atropine-induced changes in spontaneous electroencephalogram in human volunteers. Military Medicine 1990; 155: 166–170

9. Jones T W, McCarthy G, Tamborlane W V et al. Mild hypoglycemia and impairment of brain stem and cortical evoked potentials in healthy subjects. Diabetes 1990; 39(12): 1550–1555
10. Rampil I. J, Mason P, Singh H. Anesthestic potency is independent of forebrain structures in the rat. Anesthesiology 1993; 78: 707–712
11. Rampil I. J, Laster M J. No correlation between quantitative electroencephalographic measurements and movement response to noxious stimuli during isoflurane anesthesia in rats. Anesthesiology 1992; 77: 920–925
12. Franks N P, Lieb W R. Molecular and cellular mechanisms of general anaesthesia. Nature 1994; 367: 607–614
13. Genovely H, Pfeifer M A. R-R variation: The autonomic test of choice in diabetes. Diabetes/Metabolism Reviews 1988; 4: 255–271
14. Donchin Y, Feld J M, Porges S W. Respiratory sinus arrhythmia during recovery from isoflurane-nitrous oxide anaesthesia. Anesth Analg 1985; 64: 811–815
15. Porges S W. Method and apparatus for evaluating rhythmic oscillations in aperiodic physiological response systems. US Patent No. 4510944: 1985
16. Pomfrett C J D. Depth of Anaesthesia Monitoring. UK/International Patent Publication Number WO 92/06632, PCT No. GB91/01807: 1991
17. Bolshov V M, Vionor V E, Kletskin S Z et al. Method for controlling the level of anaesthesia in surgery and apparatus for effecting same. US Patent No. 3946725: 1976
18. Hrushesky W J M. Medical Instrument for noninvasive measurement of cardio-vascular characteristics. US Patent No. 4519395: 1985
19. Weinberg C R, Pfeifer M A. An improved method for measuring heart-rate variability: assessment of cardiac autonomic function. Biometrics 1984; 40: 855–861
20. Clarke B F, Ewing D J, Campbell I W. Diabetic autonomic neuropathy. Diabetologica 1979; 17: 195–212
21. Latson T W. Principles and applications of heart rate variability analysis. In: Lynch C (ed) Clinical Cardiac Electrophysiology: Perioperative Considerations. Lippincott, Philadelphia, 1994: pp 307–349
22. Kandel E R, Schwartz J H, Jessell T M. Principles of neural science, 3rd edn. Elsevier, New York, 1991
23. Smith S E, Smith S A. Heart rate variability in healthy subjects measured with a bedside computer-based technique. Clini Sci 1981; 61: 379–383
24. Jaffe R S, Fung D L. Constructing a heart-rate variability analysis system. J Clin Monit 1994; 10: 45–48
25. Hayano J, Sakakibara Y, Yamada A et al. Accuracy of assessment of cardiac vagal tone by heart rate variability in normal subjects. Am J Cardiol 1991; 67(2): 199–204
26. Kotrly K J, Ebert T, Vucins E et al. Baroreceptor reflex control of heart rate during isoflurane anaesthesia in humans. Anesthesiology 1984; 60: 173–179
27. Scheffer G J, Ten Voorde B J, Karemaker J M et al. Effects of thiopentone, etomidate, and propofol on beat-to-beat cardiovascular signals in man. Anaesthesia 1993; 48: 849–855
28. Kato M, Komatsu T, Kimura T et al. Spectral analysis of heart rate variability during isoflurane anaesthesia. Anesthesiology 1992; 77: 669–674
29. Komatsu T, Kimura T, Shimada Y. Continuous, on-line, real-time spectral analysis of heart rate variations during anaesthesia. In: Computing & Monitoring in Anaesthesia & Intensive Care. Springer-Verlag, Berlin, 1992: pp 335–338
30. Porges S W. Vagal mediation of respiratory sinus arrhythmia. Implications for drug delivery. Ann New York Acad Sci 1991; 618: 57–66
31. Pomfrett C J D, Barrie J A, Healy T E J. Respiratory sinus arrhythmia: An index of light anaesthesia. Br J Anaesth 1993; 71: 212–217
32. Pomfrett C J D, Barrie J R, Healy T E J. Respiratory sinus arrhythmia reflects surgical stimulation during light enflurane anaesthesia. Anesth Analg 1994; 78: S344
33. Latson T W, O'Flaherty D. Effects of surgical stimulation on autonomic reflex function: assessment by changes in heart rate variability. Br J Anaesth 1993; 70: 301–305

34. Pomfrett C J D, Sneyd J R, Barrie J R, Healy T E J . Respiratory sinus arrhythmia: comparison with EEG indices during isoflurane anaesthesia at 0.65 and 1.2 MAC. Br J Anaesth 1994; 72: 397–402
35. Healy T E J, Bellman M H, Pomfrett C J D. Respiratory sinus arrhythmia indicates light anaesthesia during Caesarean section. Anesth Analg 1994; 78: S156

7

Postoperative nausea and vomiting

A. Matson, M. Palazzo

A recent nationwide survey in 161 UK hospitals found a 36% incidence of postoperative nausea and vomiting (PONV) during the first 24 hours.[1] When scaled up for the UK as a whole it may be estimated that over one million patients annually suffer with PONV. The incidence of PONV from historical data suggests wide variation from 20–80%, some of which may be accounted for by study design and patient differences.[2] Although the incidence of postoperative nausea and vomiting may not have changed greatly over the past 50 years, clinical observations suggest that the severity of symptoms has.[3] However, this change should be welcomed with caution since many find persistent nausea more distressing than one or two episodes of vomiting.

In a recent study by Orkin, approximately three-quarters of the patients questioned rated freedom from nausea and vomiting as their most important postoperative requirement.[4] Patients were willing to accept dysphoria, loss of mental acuity and increased pain, in order to avoid nausea and vomiting. In a recent questionnaire analysis, nausea was second only to failure to wake up as a reason for fear of general anaesthesia.[5] Although unpleasant and embarrassing, PONV may occasionally lead to significant morbidity from dehydration, electrolyte imbalance and aspiration of vomitus. Surgical complications such as abdominal wound dehiscence, bleeding beneath skin flaps and loss of vitreous fluid following intraocular surgery may all follow severe PONV.

There are also economic implications of PONV particularly with the increasing tendency to day care surgery (60% of surgery in the USA and up to 30% of surgery in Europe). PONV resulting in an unanticipated admission leads to extra cost associated with nursing care, which may offset the cost savings of performing day care surgery.[6] Indeed PONV is cited as the most important factor in determining length of stay after ambulatory surgery and is one of the most frequent reasons for overnight admission.[7-9] The total annual cost of PONV to an average US day care centre has been estimated to be between $253 270 and $1 519 617 which could have been used to perform between 96 and 576 more surgical procedures per year.[10] The additional time spent in recovery due to PONV has been estimated at 18–61 minutes, which has an obvious impact on patient throughput. [6,10]

PONV also has economic implications for the day care patient. Patients may experience nausea and vomiting for up to 24 hours. There is consequently a significant incidence of symptoms while the patient is at home. It is not surprising then that a pilot study by the Glaxo company found that 16% of day case patients with PONV missed work the following day. What is more, carers of these patients also missed work. On average half-a-day's work was missed by both groups. [10]

WHAT SHOULD BE THE CURRENT AIM OF RESEARCH IN PONV?

Many factors have over the years been associated with an increased incidence of PONV. Most modern studies have been conducted with small numbers of patients and have failed to take complete account of the multifactorial aetiology of PONV in patient randomization. For example some studies have failed to indicate the incidence of a previous history of PONV. Although factors have been identified, little attempt has been made to weight their importance either alone or in combination. Estimation of the significance of these factors is made more difficult when current PONV research is driven by the pharmaceutical industry whose interest is primarily focussed on new antiemetics. New drugs may reduce PONV compared with placebo, but PONV rates of 15–20% although statistically significant is hardly progress. The aim should be clinical significance with rates at zero. The current unstructured hit-and-miss approach of testing a new drug against either placebo or an established old drug is unlikely to make any useful advance towards the goal of a zero incidence of PONV. It would appear that a new approach is required in which factor identification, their weights and quantification of risk is the basis upon which targetted preventive therapy is given. This needs a well-designed large observational study on a scale similar to those of Waters in 1936 and Dent in 1955. [11,12] Risk stratification would allow studies to estimate risk benefit analysis for routine antiemetic prophylaxis. In addition multiple antiemetic therapy should be explored as a potential method for dealing with PONV. It is surprising that although it is accepted that the causes of PONV are multifactorial, there has been no clinical examination in anaesthesia (unlike post chemotherapy emesis) of drug combinations. It is possible that very low doses of two or three agents given together may be more efficacious with less side effects. Such data would lead to informed clinical decisions such as which patients should receive routine prophylaxis, which drug or combination and what is the likelihood of achieving 0% PONV. It is likely that with a goal of zero for PONV the use of antiemetics will rise.

Some attempt has been made to re-examine the risk factors and weight their importance by Palazzo and Evans. In their small study the design was limited to specifically isolate patient factors such as sex, age, weight, anxiety, past medical history of PONV or motion sickness, etc. The study also included an evaluation of the impact of postoperative opiates. Table 7.1 summarizes their findings. The anaesthetic was deliberately standardized and the surgery confined to simple orthopaedic procedures so that factors related to the type of anaesthesia and surgery had no variance and could not contribute to analysis.[13] This study, however, needs to be repeated on a larger scale to include anaesthetic and surgical factors so that their relative impact compared to the patient factors can be assessed.

As yet, we have only a limited understanding of why some patients vomit whereas others remain symptom free. A brief review of the physiology of PONV and its causative factors follows.

Table 7.1 The comparative risk of PONV in the first 24 hours after surgery in patients having undergone orthopaedic procedures (derived from a prospective logistic regression analysis of patient factors)

Fixed patient factors	Probability of postoperative sickness* (%)
Males	1
Males receiving postoperative opiates	5.6
Females	6.7
Males with a previous history of PONV (PMH)	25.7
Females receiving postoperative opiates	40.3
Females with PMH and receiving postoperative opiates	59.3
Males with PMH and receiving postoperative opiates	76.4

Adapted from Palazzo and Evans 1993.[13]
* Vomiting, nausea and retching in the first postoperative 24 hours

SUMMARY OF THE PHYSIOLOGY OF VOMITING

Nausea is an unpleasant sensation associated with the desire to vomit or the feeling that vomiting is imminent. Vomiting is the forceful expulsion of upper gastrointestinal contents from the mouth and is usually preceded by retching. These reflexes presumably developed to protect the body from the effects of ingested toxins and discourage further intake.[14]

The main sensors of emetic stimuli are located in the gut and the chemoreceptor trigger zone (CRTZ). The emetic stimuli in the gut are detected by two types of vagal afferent fibres:

- Mechanoreceptors, located in the muscular wall of the gut and activated by contraction and distension of the gut or physical damage.
- Chemoreceptors located in the mucosa of the upper gut monitor the intraluminal environment and respond to noxious substances.

The CRTZ lies within the area postrema of the brain stem.[15] The area postrema is able to detect circulating toxins in the blood or cerebrospinal fluid (CSF). Stimulation of either the gastrointestinal afferents or the CRTZ will activate the vomiting centre in the medulla.[14] Afferent impulses from other areas can also influence the vomiting centre, notably the vestibular labyrinthine system which is essential for induction of motion sickness. Studies in man have shown that labyrinthine stimulation can influence the emetic response to apomorphine.[16]

There is little doubt that inputs from higher centres such as the limbic system and visual cortex can induce nausea and vomiting, but the magnitude of their role is unclear. Interestingly, Williams in a recent study found a reduction in the incidence of vomiting from 69% to 32% when patients were exposed to positive intraoperative suggestions regarding PONV.[17]

FACTORS ASSOCIATED WITH AN INCREASED INCIDENCE OF PONV

Traditionally the factors associated with PONV have been conveniently divided into those related to the patient, the anaesthetic and the surgery. However, in practice the anaesthetist and the surgeon are faced with only some factors which they can alter (variable factors) the remainder being predetermined by the patient, such as sex or the type of operation being undertaken (fixed factors). A short review follows of fixed and variable factors.

Fixed factors

These factors are predominantly patient determined and may be divided between those in which the association with PONV is strong and those in which the association is weak.

Weak associations; age, weight and anxiety

The largest studies suggest that the incidence of PONV in adults decreases with increasing age.[18,19] In his survey, Cohen analysed interview data from 16 000 postoperative patients at four teaching hospitals and found an increased relative risk for PONV of 1.36 for patients less than 50 years old when compared with persons more than 70 years old.[18]

The incidence of PONV in children is less clear. Vance, in a study of 457 patients, found the rate of PONV in children under 12 to be twice that in adults (39% vs 18%).[20] However, there is evidence from Rowley and Brown that the incidence of PONV decreased in children aged under three (20–30% in the first 18 hours after surgery) when compared with those aged between 3 and puberty (42–51%).[21] Unfortunately, it is not clear whether this difference is related to premedication. Further uncertainty in the true trend of the incidence of PONV follows the finding by Patel and Hannallah in a survey of 4998 children day cases which revealed a rate of vomiting higher in 1–2 year olds compared with 4-year-olds.[9]

Equally variable data exists for the relationship between PONV and obesity. Although it is clear that obesity may alter anaesthetic management, it is difficult to separate the latter from a specific effect of fatness on PONV. The most obvious change in anaesthetic management is the tendency to prolong mask ventilation to maintain good gas exchange while preparing for intubation. Several authors have suggested that the increased incidence of PONV in obese patients is because adipose tissue acts as a reservoir for inhaled anaesthetic agent and that these agents are the significant causative factor.[22,23] More recently, a large, controlled trial found no relationship between body mass index and PONV.[24] In this latter study chest inflation using a simple face mask was avoided. The absence of relationship between weight and PONV is supported by Cohen's large survey and the study by Palazzo and Evans on fixed risk factors.[13,18]

It has been suggested that anxiety prior to anaesthesia and surgery is associated with an increase in nausea and vomiting although Palazzo and Evans were unable to isolate this as a significant factor in their prospective study.[13] Quinn found a highly significant association between preoperative anxiety and postoperative nausea after general anaesthesia, but no relationship was seen between anxiety and vomiting.[19] The mechanism might be related to catecholamine-induced delayed gastric emptying or a central emetogenic effect.[25,26]

Strong associations; sex, past medical history

There is considerable evidence that adult females patients experience more PONV than males. The increase has been estimated as between 2–4 times that of males.[18,19,22,23,27,28] When the type of operation and anaesthetic was standardized among males and females, Palazzo and Evans were able to demonstrate a more than sixfold increase in PONV risk for females compared with males.[13] This relative risk was further increased if the males and females had received opiates. However, inclusion of a past anaesthetic history of PONV resulted in a surprising levelling of risk between males and females. The suggestion from this work is that although females appear to have an indigenous increased risk of PONV, postoperative opiates and a previous history of PONV may be far more important and are able to overwhelm the effect of sex, reducing the difference between sexes. Thus in any study some consideration must be given to the make up of the patient cohort, not so much on the ratios of males to females or the numbers who have a past history of emesis, but more on the combination of risk factors in the individuals. To avoid bias in selection it has been suggested that individual risks for patients should be calculated and the mean of these risks computed for the groups being compared.[13] The only other way to avoid such unbalancing of risks between groups is by use of extremely large numbers.

The difference between males and females might be explained by endocrine changes. It is notable that no sex difference is observed in prepubertal children or the elderly.[21,29] Honkavaara and colleagues examined the influence of the menstrual cycle on PONV and found that the need for antiemetics was highest in the luteal phase.[30] These results contrast with those of Beattie and colleagues who in a retrospective study found a fourfold increase in the risk of PONV in patients menstruating at the time of surgery.[31] However, in a second prospective study, he found maximum PONV when surgery was performed on days 25–4 of the menstrual cycle.[32] Coburn and colleagues in a study of 504 patients found an association between the risk of vomiting and peak plasma oestradiol levels and the patient's expectation of vomiting based on previous experience of anaesthesia.[33]

Most anaesthetists would consider that patients who have previously suffered emesis with anaesthesia are at increased risk with a subsequent anaesthetic. It may be difficult to make a retrospective assessment of the trigger factors present at the time of a previous anaesthetic, particularly if the anaesthetic notes are incomplete or unavailable. Most studies suggest an increased risk of PONV up to three times in patients who have experienced previous PONV.[27,28,34] Palazzo and Evans found that the risk of PONV varied depending on whether the patient was male or female and whether they had been given postoperative opiates. Females with a past history had a twofold increase in risk (from 6.7 to 13.5%) of PONV when compared with females with no previous history. However the risk increased over eightfold (6.7 to 59.3%) when females with no history were compared with females with a past history who also received postoperative opiates. Males on the other hand have a very low baseline risk; 1% compared with females (6.7%), but those males with a previous history of PONV increased their risk to over 25% and this rose to 76% when postoperative opiates were also given (Table 7.1). Therefore, the impact of additional risk factors for PONV in males appears to be far more significant than in females.

Other patient factors

Patients with intra-abdominal pathology or raised intracranial pressure, swallowing blood or with full stomachs are at increased risk of postoperative emesis.[3] Smokers seem to have a higher propensity to PONV.[18]

Variable factors

Unlike fixed factors, variable factors may be modified to some extent by the anaesthetist and surgeon. The extent to which modification of these factors influences PONV outcome depends on the relative impact of these factors compared to any pre-existing fixed factors. In a prospective evaluation of a logistic regression model for prediction of nausea and vomiting the outcome of more than 70% of patients could be correctly predicted based on fixed factors alone.[35] This suggests that there may be relatively little additional impact due to variable factors. The variable factors of interest are those related to the choice and conduct of anaesthesia and surgery.

The anaesthetist

As early as 1960 Bellville noted that the rate of PONV was higher when the anaesthetic was administered by an inexperienced anaesthetist.[22] The explanation proffered was that inexperienced anaesthetists tended to maintain deeper levels of anaesthesia. Hovorka and colleagues have recently shown that the rate of PONV is indeed related to the experience of the anaesthetist and the effect persisted for up to 6 hours postoperatively.[36] It is assumed that these findings were due to differences in the vigour and extent of gaseous inflation of the stomach, although there was no evidence for this. Interestingly, the rate of PONV is reduced by perioperative gastric aspiration and in one study gastric aspiration actually increased the incidence of PONV.[37,38]

Anaesthetic technique – local anaesthesia

Although there are no prospective studies comparing the incidence of nausea and vomiting after spinal and general anaesthesia, it is generally assumed that spinal anaesthesia alone is associated with a lower incidence of PONV than general anaesthesia, providing complications such as hypotension and high block are avoided. The overall incidence of PONV following spinal anaesthesia has been reported to range from 13–42%.[39]

Carpenter and colleagues recently undertook a prospective study of 952 patients undergoing spinal anaesthesia for a variety of procedures in which they found the incidence of nausea and vomiting was 18% and 7% respectively.[40] They found that the highest incidence of PONV was associated with use of procaine. The occurrence of PONV was also associated with high spinal blockade, a resting heart rate of greater than 60 and hypotension (systolic pressure of less than 80 mmHg).

Ratra and colleagues in a much earlier study also found that intraoperative hypotension (less than 80 mmHg systolic) was associated with PONV but were able to reduce this by the administration of 100% oxygen; they suggested that hypoxia of the vomiting centre may contribute to emesis.[41] The administration of atropine reduces the incidence of nausea and vomiting associated with spinal anaesthesia suggesting that unopposed vagal tone may also play a role.[2]

Regional anaesthesia is associated with an even lower incidence of intra and postoperative emesis.[19] Dent in a prospective study found a 4.3% incidence of emesis after peripheral nerve block compared with 11.1% after spinal, whereas Bonica's group found an incidence of 8.8% associated with local anaesthesia of the limbs.[11,42]

Anaesthetic technique – general anaesthesia

The conduct of a general anaesthetic is largely based on personal preference. Anaesthetists vary in their use of Guedel airways, nasogastric tubes, frequency of mouth suction, mask inflation of the lungs, intubation rates, placement of laryngeal masks and the use of spontaneous or controlled ventilation. There has not been a detailed prospective study of these variables but the authors suspect that their influence is likely to be smaller than the choice of drugs. There has been some considerable examination of the effect of anaesthetic drugs on PONV; some of these will now be discussed.

Anaesthetic drugs

Opioids

By far the most important group of drugs to influence PONV are the opioids; their effects overwhelm any minor differences between individual inhalational agents. Unfortunately opioid analgesia is almost mandatory for any operation even if only given as part of premedication. In a well designed study, Riding demonstrated in patients undergoing ERPC an increase in PONV from 22.4% in controls to 66.7% in patients receiving premedication with 10 mg morphine. The addition of atropine in the premedication reduced the incidence of nausea and vomiting to 35.2%.[43]

Numerous studies have attempted to compare the relative emetic effect of different opioids.[22,27,44] It would appear that the majority of opioids are equally emetogenic, although the incidence of PONV may be greater with buprenorphine.[45-47] Unfortunately there is also some evidence that avoidance of opioids may also result in PONV and that treatment of pain after abdominal surgery with opioids may reduce the incidence of nausea.[48] Quinn found an association between mean pain score and incidence of nausea and vomiting.[19] Palazzo and Evans in their quantification of risk factors found that the risk of PONV increased over fivefold when postoperative opioid analgesia was included.[13]

Induction agents

Unlike opioids where alternative preparations do not appear to result in differences in the incidence of PONV, individual induction agents do seem to have a variable impact. This is not surprising considering their differing chemical origins. Of the currently available induction agents etomidate and methohexitone are associated with higher rates of PONV than thiopentone.[49] Ketamine is thought to increase the incidence of PONV, but there are no well-controlled studies to support this.[2]

The most significant recent advance has been the widespread use of propofol for inductions, which is associated with a lower incidence of PONV.[50] Numerous prospective studies support this finding.[51,52] When propofol is also used for maintenance of anaesthesia the incidence of PONV is reported to be even lower.[8,53,54] In children, Martin and his colleagues found a much lower rate of PONV among patients induced and maintained with propofol (18%) compared with those induced and maintained with halothane (34%).[55]

The reduced occurrence of PONV associated with the use of propofol has led some to suggest that propofol may possess direct antiemetic properties. Borgeat and colleagues, in a prospective study, treated patients with severe postoperative vomiting using subhypnotic bolus doses of propofol and achieved a large reduction in PONV compared with placebo (81% vs. 35%).[56] Unfortunately, patients successfully treated had a 28% relapse rate within the first 30 minutes of therapy (22% for placebo). The mechanism of this antiemetic effect remains to be explained.

Inhalational agents

Older volatile agents such as ether and cyclopropane caused a very high rate of PONV which was thought to be due to high concentrations of circulating catecholamines. The inhalational agents in widespread use today, namely isoflurane, enflurane and halothane are associated with lesser degrees of PONV.[57]

Tracey and colleagues compared halothane, enflurane and isoflurane in 75 female patients undergoing minor gynaecological surgery and found that nausea occurred in 8, 12 and 32% of patients respectively in the first 24 hours postoperatively.[58] Conversely, Hovorka and colleagues in a study of 180 patients found that isoflurane was associated with less emetic sequelae than enflurane in the first 2 postoperative hours but at 24 hours there was no difference in the two groups.[59] A large retrospective analysis of 17 201 patients revealed a similar incidence of PONV for all three agents.[60] It would therefore appear that any differences between these three volatile agents are small and of no clinical significance. Preliminary information on desflurane and sevoflurane suggests that use is associated with a similar rate of PONV as the other volatile agents.[2]

A review suggested that N_2O might have a significant role in the incidence of PONV but there was very little prospective data to support this.[3] Several studies since have tried to clarify the role of nitrous oxide in this area and it would seem on balance that N_2O probably does contribute to PONV. In general, those studies that support an emetic effect have been in patients undergoing minor surgery of short duration.[53,61-63] Reports finding no association with PONV have generally been in patients who have undergone more serious surgery requiring postoperative opioid analgesia.[28,64-68] Unfortunately in these studies it is difficult to determine whether there was a genuine lack of effect of N_2O or whether the opiates overwhelmed what may have been a postive but weak nitrous oxide effect.

There have been four proposed mechanisms for N_2O induced emesis; actions on central opioid receptors,[61] changes in middle ear pressure,[61] sympathetic nerve stimulation[25] and gastrointestinal distension.[3] Changes in middle ear pressure was recently ruled out as a mechanism by Russell and colleagues who examined the tympanic membrane of an individual experiencing nausea and vomiting following hyperbaric N_2O anaesthesia.[69] Gastric distension secondary to nitrous oxide diffusion is probably not as impotant as the gastric distension that occurs by mask support of ventilation at the beginning of anaesthesia. Recently, Murakawa and colleagues measured various neurotransmitters in the brains of rats following exposure to N_2O and found evidence of activation of mesocortical and medullary periventricular dopaminergic systems during the initial 2 hours of exposure.[70] These changes subsided after 4 hours of exposure, suggesting an acute tolerance phenomenon.

Neuromuscular blockade

Neuromuscular blockade with nondepolarizing drugs is not thought to affect the incidence of PONV, however, reversal of neuromuscular block with neostigmine may. Two recent studies have shown an increase in the rate of PONV associated with the reversal of atracurium and mivacurium.[71,72] In another study by Boeke, however, no significant difference in PONV could be found between reversed and unreversed patients, although there was a lower requirement for antiemetic therapy in the group who received neostigmine.[73] The difference in results might be explained by the lower dose of neostigmine used in these two recent studies.

Other anaesthetic factors

Other factors such as hypoxaemia, hypotension, and early ingestion of food, have been implicated in PONV but few have been isolated as significant. Comroe and Dripps noted a close relationship between morphine use and PONV after movement and observed that this effect could last for several hours.[74] This may be a large factor in the development of PONV after dischange from day surgery units. Kamath and colleagues found that 66% of patients who identified a cause for PONV blamed movement.[75] These patients tended to have a susceptibility to motion sickness.

Surgery

Unlike anaesthetic technique which can be very varied, the type of surgery needed by an individual patient could be considered a fixed factor in the same way as patient age and sex. This of course is now changing with the increased choice between open and laparoscopic surgical techniques. A recent survey showed a considerable difference in the incidence of PONV among surgical specialities (Table 7.2). However, it is unclear if the type of surgery dictates the anaesthetic technique. If so the anaesthetic may have the greater influence on PONV. Gynaecological laparoscopic surgery has an incidence of PONV between 50 and 60% similar to open upper

Table 7.2   Incidence of PONV in the first 24 hours after surgery

Incidence of PONV (%)	Surgical speciality
42	Gynaecology
41	Orthopaedics
40	Cardiothoracic
36	ENT
36	General Surgery
26	Urology
13	Ophthalmology
36	Overall

Adapted from a survey[1]

abdominal surgery.[60,66,69,76,77] Ear sugery also carries a high rate of PONV, 40–50%, when compared with other head and neck surgery.[1,20] It is suggested that this is related to stimulation of the auriculotemporal branch of the facial nerve (bat ear surgery) and labyrinthine pathways (middle ear surgery).[58] In the recent Medicare survey, a surprisingly high incidence of PONV was specifically noted in patients undergoing laminectomy (67%), mitral valve replacement (67%) and kidney procedures (63%).[1]

In children, the surgical case mix associated with high rates of nausea and vomiting is different. Strabismus surgery is associated with a PONV rate of 40–80% in children over 2 years old.[26,58] Speculation on the cause of emesis in this procedure includes stimulation of the 'oculoemetic' reflex during traction on the extraocular muscles and visual image distortion. Traction on the inferior oblique muscle is especially associated with PONV presumably because this muscle is least accessible and is therefore subjected to the greatest degree of traction. The theory of visual image distortion is not supported by a reduction in PONV rate by covering one eye.[26]

Adenotonsillectomy is also associated with a high PONV rate in children (36–76%).[9,21,78,79] This is thought to be due to the irritant effect of blood on the oesophagogastric chemoreceptors, irritation of trigeminal afferents during surgery and opioid administration.[26] Superficial procedures carry a lower rate of PONV in children.[21,42]

MANAGEMENT OF PONV

Ideally patients with a tendency to PONV would be readily predictable and therefore the condition 100% preventable. However, the level of risk for PONV would need to be balanced against the complications related to the measures taken. For example, avoidance of opiates may be possible for minor procedures such as dilatation and curettage but difficult to justify for major abdominal surgery in the absence of other analgesic techniques such as epidural or spinal anaesthesia. Equally, routine antiemetics might be considered unacceptable in a group of patients whose risk of emesis is less than 5% because of the higher incidence of side effects. Unfortunately, although the incidence of side effects from antiemetics has been examined, risk benefit analysis for routine antiemetic therapy has not been explored in patients stratified for risk of PONV. Adriani and colleagues proposed that routine antiemetics were not justified, but his patient population only had a 3.5% incidence of PONV.[80] In spite of the lack of information in this area it would seem reasonable to us that prophylaxis should always be offered, regardless of predicted risk of PONV, to patients in whom aspiration would be inevitable should they vomit. Examples of such patients are those with wired jaws.

Other than the avoidance of opiates the prevention and treatment of PONV is primarily based on antiemetic therapy and supportive care. Antiemetic therapy is based on antagonism of the four major neurotransmitter systems which play an important role in mediating the emetic response, namely, dopaminergic, histaminic, muscarinic cholinergic and $5HT_3$. A brief summary of the more popular agents follows, although further information may be obtained from a more detailed review.[81]

Metoclopramide

Metoclopramide has been used extensively in the management of PONV over the past 30 years. It has both central and peripheral antiemetic actions. Centrally it blocks dopamine at the CRTZ and peripherally it increases lower oesophageal sphincter tone and enhances gastrointestinal motility, thereby preventing the delayed gastric emptying produced by opioids.[2] Metoclopramide also has some anti $5HT_3$ effect which may contribute to its antiemetic activity especially at high doses.[82,83] Approximately half of the numerous studies investigating its efficacy have found metoclopramide to be no better than placebo.[81] This finding is probably related to the fact that metoclopramide is rapidly redistributed after intravenous administration ($T_{1/2}\alpha = 4.9$ min) and has an elimination half-life of approximately 3 to 4 hours.[84] Its effect is therefore short lived and, if given prophylactically, should be administered at the end of surgery to have a reliable effect in the early postoperative period.

The most important side effects associated with the use of metoclopramide are extrapyramidal reactions, usually of the dystonic type. Reactions tend to occur in children and young adults when doses greater than 0.5 mg/kg are used. Sedation can occur in patients on long term therapy, but is rarely a problem in relation to recovery from anaesthesia.[85] However, a significant incidence of restlessness and agitation has been reported after administration of metoclopramide 10–20 mg as premedication.[86] Cardiovascular side effects such as hypotension, tachycardia and severe bradycardia have been reported after intravenous administration of metoclopramide.

Phenothiazines

Phenothiazines are antiemetics by virtue of their ability to block dopamine receptors. Phenothiazines also have mild antihistamine, antimuscarinic and peripheral anti-5HT effects. Promethazine is still used as a premedicant because of its sedative and significant antiemetic effects. In the prevention and treatment of PONV, only prochlorperazine and perphenazine have been used extensively. Although only limited data exist on the efficacy of prochlorperazine for the prevention of PONV, this drug is the most commonly used antiemetic.[1] Prochlorperazine has been shown to be effective in the treatment of established vomiting after anaesthesia and its antiemetic effects have been shown to last for at least 4 hours.[87] Important side effects include extrapyramidal reactions, particularly in children and young adults receiving greater than 10 mg. Untoward sedation can occur after a single dose. Cardiovascular side effects namely hypotension and dysrhythmias may occur, particularly in the hypovolaemic and elderly.

Although undoubtedly an effective antiemetic, perphenazine also causes sedation and a high incidence of extrapyramidal reactions. Recently, dixyrazine has been shown to be effective in the prophylaxis and treatment of PONV following paediatric stabismus surgery.[88]

Butyrophenones

In this group of drugs, only droperidol is commonly used by anaesthetists. Again, it exerts its antiemetic effects by antagonism of dopamine receptors.[87] The majority of studies have found droperidol more effective than placebo as a prophylactic antiemetic. In those studies in which droperidol was found to be ineffective, it was administered at induction of anaesthesia.[81] Droperidol has a redistribution half-life of 10 minutes and an elimination half-life of 2 hours so it is probably best given towards the end of surgery.[89] Unfortunately, the use of droperidol is associated with frequent side effects. Drowsiness may be of significance in day care anaesthesia.[24,77,89,90] Extrapyramidal reactions may occur several hours after administration and in general occurs with doses larger than 2.5 mg intravenously (in adults), however, extrapyramidal reactions to low dose droperidol (0.65 mg) have also been reported.[91]

The most common side effect with droperidol is a feeling of anxiety and restlessness. Melnick found that following 1.25 mg of droperidol 23% of patients suffered from these feelings until the day following discharge.[91] This may also be the case with even smaller doses. The use of low dose droperidol has become popular in an attempt to reduce side effects, however it seems to be less effective for procedures associated with a high rate of emesis, e.g. strabismus surgery.[26,92]

Anticholinergics

Hyoscine and atropine are among the oldest of antiemetic agents and are traditionally given with opiate premedication principally for their drying effects. Their antiemetic efficacy has clearly been demonstrated.[43,93,94] However, the administration of hyoscine is associated with dose-dependent side

effects. A transdermal preparation of hyoscine has been developed to reduce these side effects and also to overcome the problem of its short plasma
half-life. Although the transdermal preparation is effective in prevention of
motion sickness its effectiveness for prevention of PONV seems less clear.[95]
Side effects such as dry mouth, visual disturbance and drowsiness are
relatively frequent but are minor in comparison with other antiemetics.
Hyoscine psychosis has been reported following transdermal hyoscine. This
is a risk particularly in the elderly.[96]

Antihistamines

Many antihistamines of differing chemical groups have been developed and
used for the prevention of motion sickness. Only cyclizine has been used extensively in the management of PONV. Most of the cyclizine studies have
showed it to be effective in the prevention and treatment of PONV. Although
it has side effects which include sedation and dry mouth, its advantage over
other agents is the very low incidence of extrapyramidal side effects.

5HT$_3$ antagonists

Radioligand binding studies have demonstrated a high density of 5HT$_3$
receptors in areas known to be involved in the emetic reflex, including
vagal afferent terminals in the gastrointestinal mucosa, the brain stem
dorsovagal nucleus, the nucleus solitarius and the area postrema.[97] It is
possible that anaesthetic agents may stimulate neurones within the area
postrema and activate the vomiting reflex via a 5HT mediated pathway.
The control of emesis is mediated via the 5HT$_3$ receptor subtype and various
5HT$_3$ antagonists have now been developed including ondansetron,
ganisetron and tropisetron, of which only the former has been extensively
used to date.

   Ondansetron may be administered orally or intravenously. Its plasma
half-life is 3 hours and excretion is mainly by hydroxylation in the liver.
Intramuscular ondansetron has the same bioavailability as intravenous
ondansetron. Several studies have demonstrated its efficacy in prophylaxis
and treatment of PONV in adults and children mainly when compared
with placebo.[78,98,99] It would appear that ondansetron 4 mg is the optimal
intravenous dose for the prevention and treatment of emesis and it is claimed
to be effective for a 24 hour period. Ondansetron 8 mg may confer additional
benefit in the prophylaxis of PONV in patients with a previous history of
PONV.[99] In children a dose of 0.15 mg/kg has been found to be effective.[78] A
single oral dose of ondansetron 16 mg given 1 hour prior to induction of
anaesthesia has also been found to be effective in the prophylaxis of PONV in
patients with and without a history of PONV or motion sickness.[98]

   Ondansetron so far has a good safety profile, the most important side
effects being constipation, headache and a warm sensation or flushing on

iv. administration. To date few studies have been undertaken to establish the comparative efficacy of ondansetron with older antiemetics. From the information available, it would appear that ondansetron is better than placebo and might be superior to both droperidol and metoclopramide. However, much further comparative evaluation needs to be done before it is considered to be better or more cost effective than the established alternatives, furthermore it might be too early to judge its side effect profile.

Additional therapy

Ephedrine, an indirectly acting sympathomimetic, is useful for treating nausea and vomiting secondary to hypotension in spinal anaesthesia, it is also useful in nausea developed after postural changes when attempting to mobilize post surgery.[2]

The use of acupuncture at the P6 or Neiguan point near the wrist to prevent PONV has stimulated considerable intrest. Acupuncture seems to be as successful as other conventional antiemetics in reducing nausea and vomiting after minor gynaecological procedures. Acupressure is less effective in terms of duration of effect.[100] However, failure of acupunture to influence the PONV rate has been reported after paediatric strabismus surgery and tonsillectomy.[79]

SUMMARY

Although PONV remains a problem there is a clinical perception that its severity may well have diminished. What is not clear is whether patients who in the past may have vomited now simply experience nausea. However for many patients, persistent nausea may be more distressing than a single vomit. Several factors may account for the perceived decrease in severity of PONV including the increase in day surgery, in which opioids are avoided and the observation period is shorter. But perhaps as important is the widespread use of propofol which may have inadvertently introduced an antiemetic drug into routine anaesthetic practice. In addition, there is a greater awareness of PONV and a lower threshold to starting prophylactic care.

Further progress must be towards eradicating PONV and not being content with products or methods that simply provide 'statistical significance' over placebos. As a first step, studies should be directed towards patients with a quantified risk of PONV. This should be followed by an exploration of the efficacy of multiple antiemetics in individuals. It is clear that as yet there is no magic bullet for the complete control or treatment of PONV. Once the efficacy of agents or their combinations have been established against stratified risk groups it would then be appropriate to explore the risk benefit of routine prophylactic antiemetics for these groups. These exploratory studies are now underway in our own institution and hopefully may offer better guidelines as to whom we should offer prophylaxis and what that should be. For the time being collective wisdom would suggest that attention should be paid to the factors outlined below.

KEY POINTS FOR CLINICAL PRACTICE

- Establish which patients are at high risk of PONV or in whom PONV would compromise outcome so prophylaxis may be given. Patients with a history of PONV and receiving opiates or patients with wired jaw administer prophylaxis: droperidol 1–3 mg near the termination of surgery or ondansetron 4 mg at induction.
- Induce anaesthesia with propofol, the induction agent associated with the lowest rate of PONV which may have some intrinsic antiemetic activity.
- Avoid opioids if possible by more use of NSAIDS and local anaesthetic techniques.
- Avoid sudden movement and changes in posture during recovery. Move patients slowly especially round corners.
- Early intake of food and drink postoperatively should be discouraged.
- If emesis does occur, attention should be given to hydration and pain management.
- If one antiemetic is unsuccessful a drug with a different mechanism of action should be tried. Cyclizine, perfenazine, prochlorperazine, droperidol and ondansetron should be first choice.
- At all times the patient should be reassured.

REFERENCES

1. The incidence and impact of postoperative nausea and vomiting. Medicare Audits Ltd. Survey on PONV. Synergy Medical Education. Richmond, Surrey, 1993
2. Watcha M, White P.Postoperative Nausea and Vomiting. Its Etiology, Treatment and Prevention. Anesthesiology 1992; 77: 162–184
3. Palazzo M G A, Strunin L. Anaesthesia and emesis 1. Etiology. Canad J Soc Anaesth 1984; 31: 178–187
4. Orkin F. What do patients want? Preferences for immediate postoperative recovery. Anesth Analg 1992; 74: S225
5. van Wijk M, Smallhout B. A postoperative analysis of the patient's view of anaesthesia in a Netherlands teaching hospoital. Anaesthesia 1990; 45: 679–682
6. Morris R, Ernst E, Greaves D et al. An audit of the incidence and costs associated with postoperative nausea and vomiting (PONV) following major gynecological surgery. Br Anaesth 1993; 70(suppl 1): A2
7. Gold B S, Kitz D S, Lecky J H, Neuhaus J M. Unanticipated admission to the hospital following ambulatory surgery. JAMA 1989; 262: 3008–3010
8. Green G, Jonsson L. Nausea; the most important factor determining length of stay after ambulatory anaesthesia. A comparative study of isoflurane and/or propofol techniques. Acta Anaesthesiol Scand 1993; 37: 742–746
9. Patel R, Hannallah R. Anesthetic complications following pediatric ambulatory surgery; A 3 yr study. Anesthesiology 1988; 69: 1009–1012
10. Hirsch J. Impact of postoperative nausea and vomiting in the surgical setting. Anaesthesia 1994; 49 (supplement): 30–33

11. Dent S, Ramachandra V, Stephen C R. Postoperative vomiting; incidence analysis and therapeutic measures in 3000 patients. Anesthesiology 1955; 16: 564–572
12. Waters R M. The present state of cyclopropane. BMJ 1936; 2: 1013–1017
13. Palazzo M, Evans R. Logistic regression analysis of fixed patient factors for postoperative sickness; A model for risk assessment. Br J Anaesth 1993; 70: 135–140
14. Andrews P. Physiology of nausea and vomiting. Br J Anaesth 1992; 69 (suppl 1): 2S–19S
15. Borison H, Wang S. Physiology and pharmacology of vomiting. Pharmacol Rev 1953; 5: 192–230
16. Issacs B. The influence of head and body position on the emetic action of apomorphine in man. Clin Sci 1957; 16: 215–221
17. Williams A, Hind M, Sweeney B. The incidence and severity of postoperative nausea and vomiting in patients exposed to positive intraoperative suggestions. Anaesthesia 1994; 49: 340–342
18. Cohen M, Duncan P, Deboer D, Tweed W. The postoperative interview – assessing risk factors for nausea and vomiting. Anesth Analg 1994; 78: 7–16
19. Quinn A, Brown J, Wallace P, Asbury A. Studies in postoperative sequelae. Nausea and vomiting still a problem. Anaesthesia 1994; 49: 62–65
20. Vance J, Neill R, Norris W. The incidence and aetiology of postoperative nausea and vomiting in a plastic surgical unit. Br J Plastic Surg 1973; 26: 336–339
21. Rowley M P, Brown T C. Postoperative vomiting in children. Anaesth Intens Care 1982; 10: 309–313
22. Bellville J W, Bross I D J, Howlands W S. Postoperative nausea and vomiting. IV, Factors related to postoperative nausea and vomiting. Anesthesiology 1960; 21: 186–193
23. Smessaert A, Schehr C, Artusio J. Nausea and vomiting in the immediate postanesthetic period. JAMA 1959; 170: 2072–2076
24. McKenzie R, Wadhwa R, Lim N et al. Antiemetic effectiveness of intramuscular hydroxyzine compared with intramuscular droperidol. Anesth Analg 1981; 60: 783–788
25. Jekins L, Lahay D. Central mechanisms of vomiting related to catecholamine responses; anaesthetic implications. Canad Anaesth Soc J 1971; 18: 434–441
26. Lerman J. Surgical and patient factors involved in postoperative nausea and vomiting. Br J Anaesth 1992; 69 (Suppl 1): 24S–32S
27. Burtles R, Peckett B. Postoperative vomiting. Br J Anaesth 1957; 29: 114–123
28. Muir J J, Warner M A, Offord K P et al. Role of nitrous oxide and other factors in postoperative nausea and vomiting: a randomized and blinded prospective study. Anesthesiology 1987; 66: 513–518
29. Money K, Cheung B. Another function of the inner ear; facilitation of the emetic response to poisons. Aviation Space and Environmental Medicine 1983; 54: 208–211
30. Honkavaara P, Lehtinen A-M, Hovorka J, Kortilla K. Nausea and vomiting after gynaecological laparoscopy depends on the phase of the menstrual cycle. Canad J Anaesth 1991; 38: 876–879
31. Beattie W, Lindblad T, Buckley D, Forrest J. The incidence of postoperative nausea and vomiting in women undergoing laparoscopy is influenced by the day of the menstrual cycle. Cand J Anaesth 1991; 38: 298–302
32. Beattie W, Lindblad T, Buckley D, Forrest J. Menstruation increases the risk of nausea and vomiting after laparoscopy. A prospective randomised study. Anesthesiology 1993; 78: 272–276
33. Coburn R, Lane J, Harrison K, Hennessey J. Postoperative vomiting factors in IVF patients. Aust N Z J Obstet Gynaec 1993; 33: 57–60
34. Purkis I. Factors that influence postoperative vomiting. Canad Anaesth Soc J 1964; 11: 335–353
35. Samra G, Littlejohn I, Broomhead C et al. Predicting postoperative nausea and vomiting using a logistic regression model. Br J Anaesth 1994; 72: 488P
36. Hovorka J, Korttila K, Erkola O. The experience of the person ventilating the lungs does influence postoperative nausea and vomiting. Acta Anaesthesiol Scand 1990; 34: 203–205

37. Hovorka J, Korttila K, Erkola O. Gastric aspiration at the end of anaesthesia does not decrease postoperative nausea and vomiting. Anaesth Intens Care 1990; 18: 58–61
38. Trepanier C, Isabel L. Postoperative gastric aspiration increases postoperative nausea and vomiting in outpatients. Canad J Anaesth 1993; 40: 325–358
39. Rabey P, Smith G. Anaesthetic factors contributing to postoperative nausea and vomiting. Br J Anaesth 1992; 69 (suppl 1): 40–45
40. Carpenter R, Caplan R, Brown D et al Incidence and risk factors for side effects of spinal anesthesia. Anesthesiology 1992; 76: 906–916
41. Ratra C, Badola R, Bhargava K. A study of the factors concerned in emesis during spinal anaesthesia. Br J Anaesth 1972; 44: 1208–1211
42. Bonica J J, Crepps W, Monk B, Bennett B. Postoperative nausea retching and vomiting. Anesthesiology 1958; 19: 532–540
43. Riding J E. Postoperative vomiting. J R Soc Med 1960; 53: 707–712
44. Dundee J W, Kirwan M J, Clarke R S. Anaesthesia and premedication as factors in postoperative vomiting. Acta Anaesthesiol Scand 1965; 9: 223–231
45. Fullerton T, Timm T, Kolski G, Bertino J. Prolonged nausea and vomiting associated with buprenorphine. Pharmacotherapy 1991; 11: 90–93
46. Scamman F, Ghoneim M, Korttila K. Ventilatory and mental effects of alfentanil and fentanyl. Acta Anaesthesiol Scand 1984; 28: 63–67
47. White P, Coe V, Shafer A, Sung M-L. Comparison of alfentanil with fentanyl for outpatient anesthesia. Anesthesiology 1986; 64: 99–106
48. Andersen R, Krohg K. Pain as a major cause of postoperative nausea. Canad Anaesth Soc J 1976; 23: 366–369
49. Clarke R. Nausea and vomiting. Br J Anaesth 1984; 56: 19–27
50. Borgeat A, Wilder-Smith O, Suter P. The non hypnotic therapeutic applications of propofol. Anesthesiology 1994; 80: 642–656
51. McCollum J, Milligan K, Dundee J. The antiemetic action of propofol. Anaesthesia 1988; 43: 239–240
52. Doze V, Shafer A, White P. Propofol–nitrous oxide versus thiopental–isoflurane–nitrous oxide for general anesthesia. Anesthesiology 1988; 69: 63–71
53. Watcha M, Simeon R, White P, Stevens J. Effect of propofol on the incidence of postoperative vomiting after strabismus surgery in pediatric outpatients. Anesthesiology 1991; 75: 204–209
54. Weir P, Munro H, Reynolds P et al. Propofol infusion and the incidence of emesis in pediatric outpatient strabismus surgery. Anesth Analg 1993; 76: 760–764
55. Martin T, Nicolson S, Bargas M. Propofol anesthesia reduces emesis and airway obstruction in pediatric outpatients. Anesth Analg 1993; 76: 144–148
56. Borgeat A, Wilder-Smith O, Saiah M, Rifat K. Subhypnotic doses of propofol possess direct antiemetic properties. Anesth Analg 1992; 74: 539–541
57. Kenny G. Risk factors for postoperative nausea and vomiting. Anaesthesia 1994; 49 (supplement): 6–10
58. Tracey J, Holland A, Unger L. Morbidity in minor gynaecological surgery: A comparison of halothane, enflurane and isoflurane. Br J Anaesth 1982; 54: 1213–1214
59. Hovorka J, Kortilla K, Erkola O. Nausea and vomiting after general anaesthesia with isoflurane, enflurane or fentanyl in combination with nitrous oxide and oxygen. Eur J Anaesthesiol 1988; 5: 177–182
60. Forrest J, Beattie W, Goldsmith C. Risk factors for nausea and vomiting after general anaesthesia. Can J Anaesth 1990; 37: S90
61. Melnick B, Johnson L. Effects of eliminating nitrous oxide in outpatient anesthesia. Anesthesiology 1987; 67: 982–984
62. Alexander G, Skupski J, Brown E. The role of nitrous oxide in postoperative nausea and vomiting. Anesth Analg 1984; 63: S175
63. Lonie D S, Harper N J. Nitrous oxide anaesthesia and vomiting. The effect of nitrous oxide anaesthesia on the incidence of vomiting following gynaecological laparoscopy [published erratum appears in Anaesthesia 1986 (Oct); 41: 1083]. Anaesthesia 1986; 41: 703–707

64. Kortilla K, Hovorka J, Erkola O. Nitrous oxide does not increase the incidence of nausea and vomiting after isoflurane anaesthesia. Anesth Analg 1987; 66: 761–765
65. Hovorka J, Korttila K, Erkola O. Nitrous oxide does not increase nausea and vomiting following gynaecological laparoscopy. Can J Anaesth 1989; 36: 145–148
66. Sengupta P, Plantevin O M. Nitrous oxide and day-case laparoscopy: effects on nausea, vomiting and return to normal activity. Br J Anaesth 1988; 60: 570–573
67. Sukhani R, Lurie J, Jabamoni R. Propofol for ambulatory gynaecological laparoscopy. Does omission of nitrous oxide alter postoperative emetic sequelae and recovery. Anesth Analg 1994; 78: 831–835
68. Ranta P, Nuutinen L, Laitinen J. The role of nitrous oxide in postoperative nausea and recovery in patients undergoing upper abdominal surgery. Acta Anaesthesiol Scand 1991; 35: 339–341
69. Russell G, Snider M, Richard R, Loomis J. Hyperbaric nitrous oxide as a sole anesthetic agent in humans. Anesth Analg 1990; 70: 289–295
70. Murakawa M, Adachi T, Nakao S et al Activation of the cortical and medullary dopinergic systems by nitrous oxide in rats, a possible neurochemical basis for psychotropic effects and postanesthetic nausea and vomiting. Anesth Analg 1994; 78: 376–381
71. Ding Y, Fredman B, White P. Use of mivacurium during laparoscopic surgery – effect of reversal drugs on postoperative recovery. Anesth Analg 1994; 78: 450–454
72. King M J, Milazkiewicz R, Carli F, Deacock A R. Influence of neostigmine on postoperative vomiting. Br J Anaesth 1988; 61: 403–406
73. Boeke A, Delange J, Vandruenen B, Laugemeijer J. Effect of antagonising residual neuromuscolar blockade by neostigmine and atropine on postoperative vomiting. Br J Anaesth 1994; 72: 654–656
74. Comroev J, Dripps R. Reactions to morphine in ambulatory and bed patients. Surg Gynaecol Obstet 1948; 87: 221–224
75. Kamath B, Curran J, Hawkey C et al. Anaesthesia, movement and emesis. Br J Anaesth 1990; 64: 728–730
76. Dupeyron J, Conseiller C, Levarlet M et al. The effect of oral ondansetron in the prevention of postoperative nausea and vomiting after major gynaecological surgery performed under general anaesthesia. Anaesthesia 1993; 48: 214–218
77. Madej T H, Simpson K H. Comparison of the use of domperidone, droperidol and metoclopramide in the prevention of nausea and vomiting following major gynaeco-logical surgery. Br J Anaesth 1986; 58: 884–887
78. Litman R, Catanzaro F. Ondansetron decreases emesis after tonsillectomy in children. Anesth Analg 1994; 78: 478–481
79. Yentis S, Bissonnette B. P6 acupuncture and postoperative vomiting after tonsillec-tomy in children. Br J Anaesth 1991; 67: 779–780
80. Adriani J, Summers F W, Anthony S O. Is the prophylactic use of antiemetics in surgical patients justified? JAMA 1961; 175: 666–671
81. Rowbotham D. Current management of postoperative nausea and vomiting. Br J Anaesth 1992; 69(suppl 1): 46S–59S
82. Hindle A. Recent developments in the physiology and pharmacology of 5hydroxytryptamine. Br J Anaesth 1994; 73: 395–407
83. Fozard J. Neuronal 5HT receptors in the periphery. Neuropharmacology 1984; 23: 1473–1486
84. Bateman D, Kahn C, Mashiter K, Davies D. Pharmacokinetic and concentration–effect studies with intravenous metoclopramide. Br J Clin Pharmacol 1978; 6: 401–497
85. Lind B, Breivik H. Metoclopramide and perphenazine in the prevention of postop-erative nausea and vomiting. Br J Anaesth 1970; 42: 614–617
86. Dundee J, Clarke R. The premedicant and anti-emetic action of metoclopramide. Postgrad Med J 1973; Suppl: 34–37
87. Loeser E, Bennett G, Stanley T, Machin R. Comparison of droperidol, haloperidol and prochlorperazine as postoperative antiemetics. Canad Anaesth Soc J 1979; 26: 125–127
88. Karlsson E, Larsson L, Nilsson K. The effects of prophylactic dixyrazine on

postoperative vomiting after two different anesthetic methods for squint surgery in children. Acta Anaesthesiol Scand 1993; 37: 45–48

89. Cressman W, Plostnieks J, Johnson P. Absorption, metabolism and excretion of droperidol by human subjects following intramuscular and intravenous administration. Anesthesiology 1973; 38: 363–369

90. Mortensen P T. Droperidol postoperative antiemetic effect when given intravenously to gynaecological patients. Acta Anaesthesiol Scand 1982; 26: 48–52

91. Melnick B, Sawyer R, Karambelkar D et al. Delayed side effects of droperidol after ambulatory general anesthesia. Anesth Analg 1989; 69: 748–751

92. O'Donovan N, Shaw J. Nausea and vomiting in day-case dental surgery. Anaesthesia 1984; 39: 1172–1176

93. Clarke R, Dundee J, Love W. Studies of drugs given before anaesthesia. VIII. Morphine 10 mg alone and with atropine or hyoscine. Br J Anaesth 1965; 37: 772–777

94. Dundee J, Moore J, Clarke R. Studies of drugs given before anaesthesia. V. Pethidine alone and with atropine or hyoscine. Br J Anaesth 1964; 36: 703–710

95. Wetchler B. Postoperative nausea and vomiting in day case surgery. Br J Anaesth 1992; 69 (Suppl 1): 33S–39S

96. MacEwan G, Remick R, Noone J. Psychosis due to transdermally administered scopolamine. Canad Med Assoc J 1985; 133: 431–433

97. Naylor R, Inall F. The physiology and pharmacology of postoperative nausea and vomiting. Anaesthesia 1994; 49 (suppl): 2–5

98. Rust M, Cohen L. Single oral dose ondansetron in the prevention of postoperative nausea and emesis. Anaesthesia 1994; 49: 16–23

99. Pearman M. Single dose intravenous ondansetron in the prevention of postoperative nausea and vomiting. Anaesthesia 1994; 49 (Suppl): 11–15

100. Dundee J, McMillan C. Positive evidence for P6 acupuncture antiemesis. Postgrad Med J 1991; 67: 417–422

8

Paediatric pain relief

L. J. Murdoch   J. N. Cashman

> It is our responsibility to treat pain in neonates and infants as effectively
> as we do in other patients[1]

Pain is a protective mechanism designed to alert the body to potentially injurious stimuli. The International Association for the Study of Pain has defined pain as 'an unpleasant sensory and emotional experience, associated with actual or potential tissue damage'.[2] The alleviation of pain has been the focus of continuing human effort. However, it has been recognized for some time that the management of acute pain, especially postoperative pain, has been consistently and systematically inadequate. Numerous published articles have highlighted the poor quality of the provision of postoperative pain relief in adult patients, culminating in the publication of the report commissioned jointly by the Royal College of Surgeons and the (as was then) College of Anaesthetists.[3] The report of the Joint College Working Party on Pain after Surgery, which was primarily concerned with analgesia in adult patients but did also consider paediatric patients, makes a number of recommendations including the systematic assessment and recording of postoperative pain. If anything the situation in children has been even worse; children have long been undermedicated for acute pain.[4] The report by the Audit Commission 'Children First'[5] outlines proposals for continuous audit to assess the quality of overall care delivered to children in hospital. Pain relief is one of the 10 proposed quality indicators. Fortunately, attitudes to treating pain in infants have changed dramatically during the past 15 years.[6] Nevertheless as recently as 1987 one author was prompted to write that 'it is unconscionable to continue to neglect the safe application of analgesics in our youngest patients'.[7]

There is a large body of evidence that pain is undertreated in children, particularly in neonates and infants.[8–13] The reasons for witholding analgesia are many and diverse, including:

- A difficulty in distinguishing pain from hunger or fear in preverbal children
- The myth that because some children do not act as if they are in pain, then they cannot be in pain

- The notion that children do not respond to pain to the same degree as adults
- A lack of information regarding the safety and efficacy of analgesics in young children
- An excessive concern regarding the increased risk of opioid-induced respiratory depression in children
- A fear of opioid addiction

For their part, children learn quickly that if they complain of pain then further pain, in the form of an intramuscular injection, will follow. But because the analgesic effect of the injection takes some time the child does not link the relief of the former with the latter.[14]

Over the last ten years there has been a substantial increase in our understanding and management of paediatric pain resulting in an abundance of therapeutic modalities now available to prevent and treat pain in children. It is now generally accepted that acute postoperative pain management is an integral part of the practice of paediatric anaesthesia. This review considers recent developments in the application of analgesic techniques for neonates, infants and children in acute pain.

THE DEVELOPMENT OF PAIN MECHANISMS

Pain is subjective and therefore it cannot be proven that babies feel pain. However, there is unequivocable evidence that nociceptive pathways are present even in preterm infants,[15] and that stimulation of these pathways results in behavioural, physiological, metabolic and hormonal changes consistent with pain.[15-18] Nociception is associated with signs of distress even in newborn infants.[19] The density of nociceptive nerve endings in the skin of newborn infants is similar to, or greater than, that in adults. The lack of myelination of peripheral nerves, which will slow conduction velocity, is offset almost completely by the shorter interneurone and neuromuscular distances travelled by nerve impulses. By the 24th–30th week of gestation, pain pathways to the brain stem and thalamus are completely myelinated.[14,15] Substance P and its receptors are detectable in the fetal dorsal horn at 12 to 14 weeks of gestation. Endogenous opioids are present in the plasma and cerebrospinal fluid of term infants and concentrations of beta-endorphin increase in response to stress. In addition, in the human fetus development of endogenous opioid receptors occurs in utero.[20] Sensation, as implied by cortical responses to visual and auditory stimuli, is present in preterm infants. In vivo measurements of cerebral glucose utilization have shown that the maximal rates of metabolic activity occur in sensory areas of the neonatal brain. In neonates acute painful stimuli such as circumcision and heel prick result in increases in heart rate, respiratory rate, blood pressure and palmar sweating, and a fall in transcutaneous oxygen tension. These changes can be attenuated by providing effective analgesia. Surgery results in major hormonal changes, notably increases in plasma concentrations of adrenaline, noradrenaline, insulin, glucagon, cortisol and aldosterone. The hormonal stress response can be reduced by the provision of adequate analgesia. Furthermore, complex behavioural responses seen following circumcision are abolished when local anaesthesia is used. In summary, there is a well-defined pathway for the sensation of pain in the newborn infant. A more detailed description is to be found in the comprehensive review by Anand and Hickey.[15]

Although basic somatosensory pathways are formed by birth there is considerable postnatal development in relation to pain pathways. Input from nociceptors may produce responses in the central nervous system (CNS). However, the CNS may not always be sufficiently organized to produce predictable behavioural reactions. Also, there is a lack of descending and segmental inhibition in the neonatal spinal cord resulting in less endogenous control of noxious inputs. Therefore, noxious inputs may have an even more profound effect than in adults, but the reactions will be more diffuse and the effects potentially underrated. Fitzgerald[21] provides a detailed description of the development of pain mechanisms.

PAIN TRANSMISSION

Tissue injury, such as occurs with surgical intervention, is associated with the release of numerous inflammatory mediators. Acute pain reflects the activation of nociceptors by noxious stimuli. These peripheral sensory receptors transmit information signalling acute injury along afferent A delta and C nerve fibres which project to the central nervous system (CNS). Spinal and supraspinal centres within the CNS both process and react to the information resulting from noxious stimuli. Endogenous modulation of the painful sensation can occur. Descending inhibition from supraspinal centres has an important role in modulation of pain traffic at the spinal level. There have been many excellent reviews on the neurophysiology of postoperative pain including the comprehensive reviews by Besson and Chaouch[22] and by Woolf.[23]

ASSESSMENT OF PAIN

Many factors will influence the child's response to pain. The difficulty of assessing and measuring children's pain, due to developmental, emotional and cognitive differences between adults and children, has in part been responsible for the undertreatment of their pain. Pain assessment in children relies either on objective methods (observation of physiological and behavioural changes) or subjective methods (self-assessment). Observational assessment is inferior to self assessment but is frequently the only method available in younger children.[24]

Physiological variables have been investigated as measures of pain severity. However, there are no physiological responses that directly reflect a child's perception of pain. The assessment of physiological parameters, theoretically, should provide an objective measure of pain, but it is not clear whether the responses initiated by a noxious stimulus actually correlate with pain. Adaptation rapidly occurs and autonomic responses return to normal. Anand and Hickey[15] have analysed pain and its effects, particularly physiological changes, in the neonate.

Another method of assessing and measuring children's pain relies on observation of behaviour. Behaviours commonly associated with pain include facial expression (e.g. grimace), posture (e.g. guarding), and vocalization (e.g. cry or ouch). In infants these reactions are complex and vary with age, prior state of arousal and behaviour. Nevertheless several scoring systems, based on observation of these parameters, exist including the Infant Pain Behaviour Rating Scale (IPBRS).[25] Recently more complex scoring systems, relying on observation of a greater number of parameters, have been employed to assess pain and analgesia associated with venepuncture[26] and analgesia in mechanically ventilated newborn babies.[27] In older children a number of scales have been developed and validated, including the Procedural Behaviour Rating Scale-revised (PBRS-r),[28,29] originally developed for paediatric oncology procedures, and the Children's Hospital of Eastern Ontario Pain Scale (CHEOPS),[30] devised for assessing postoperative pain.

The assessment of a child's subjective experience is the best method of obtaining information about their pain. Most children over three years of age are able to understand the concept of hurt and that there are varying degrees of hurt. The simplest, most accurate method of self report of pain intensity is the Visual Analogue Scale (VAS), where the patient scores his or her pain on a line with end points 'no pain' and 'worst pain imaginable'. The VAS has provided sensitive and reproducible results with children older than six or seven years of age. However, below this age, children have not usually developed the cognitive skills necessary for use of this system. Amongst the methods of self-report available to younger children are: the Smiley Analogue Scale,[31] in which the child is asked to select from a series of pictures of faces the one face that depicts how he or she feels at that moment. Hester's Poker Chip Tool,[32] in which children quantify their pain by seeing it as pieces of hurt that can be graded from one to four and the colour scale devised by Eland[33] where children create their own pain scale by colouring in a body outline, using different coloured crayons, which they grade from 'no hurt at all' to 'worst hurt'.

The recognition and quantification of pain are important stages in pain management. The methods of pain assessment outlined may be promising in pain research and in increasing awareness in the clinical setting of the need for analgesia, but none are without their limitations, and although one objective 'gold standard' of pain intensity would be welcomed, such a measure does not, and probably never will exist.

PAIN MANAGEMENT IN NEONATES, INFANTS AND CHILDREN

General care

Analgesic administration is but one aspect of the care of infants in pain and should be accompanied by other measures that ensure the child's comfort and minimize distress. These measures include feeding and nursing in a warm environment and contact with parents. Holding and cuddling are frequently used to pacify a baby who is upset, as are tactile stimulation, position changes and the use of dummies.[34]

Non opioid analgesic drugs

Paracetamol

This is a popular and safe analgesic in infants and neonates.[35] It is useful for the treatment of mild-to-moderate pain in a dose of 10–15 mg/kg, administered either orally or rectally, to a maximum dose of 60 mg/kg/day.

A number of studies have demonstrated erratic rectal absorption of paracetamol.[36,37] Hopkins and colleagues[36] administered paracetamol in doses ranging from 15 to 20 mg/kg, either rectally or nasogastrically, to children after cardiac surgery. In many of the children plasma paracetamol levels were inadequate for analgesia and the antipyretic effects were disappointing. The peak plasma concentration following rectal administration was lower than via the nasogastric route. These authors concluded that, because the rectal route was associated with erratic absorption of paracetamol, a dose of 20–25 mg/kg was likely to be needed. An injectable formulation of paracetamol, as the pro-drug propacetamol, exists.[38] There is limited experience of this drug, which has been used in children[39] with more studies necessary to confirm its tolerance and efficacy.

Paracetamol elimination is reduced in term neonates. The plasma elimination half-life in neonates varies between 1.2 and 4.9 hours, compared with a half-life in children of 1.4 to 3.8 hours and 1.5 to 3.0 hours in adults.[36,40] Paracetamol is excreted mainly as the glucuronide and as the sulphate, however, some drug is eliminated unchanged. Miller and colleagues[35] have suggested that infants have a reduced capacity to form the glucuronide but an increased capacity to form the sulphate. As a result the glucuronide/sulphate ratio is lower in neonates than adults, only approaching adult levels at 12 years (Table 8.1).[35] In contrast a study by Notorianni and colleagues[41] would seem to suggest that the neonate has a deficient capacity for sulphate conjugation.

Saturation of the elimination pathways following paracetamol overdose can result in toxic metabolites. However, the toxic metabolites are detoxified by glutathione which exhibits increased levels in children. This factor,

Table 8.1   Paracetamol glucuronide/sulphate ratios in neonates, children and adults[35]

	Glucuronide/sulphate ratios
Neonates	0.34
3–9 years	0.75
12 years	1.60
Adults	1.80

along with increased capacity for sulphation already referred to, is responsible for the low incidence of paracetamol hepatotoxicity in neonates.[42] There are case reports of pregnant women who have taken an overdose of paracetamol without apparent adverse effect for the fetus which has been subsequently delivered safely. In one of the largest series of its kind Riggs and colleagues[43] report on 60 pregnant women who took an overdose of paracetamol. Of 24 patients who had toxic levels of paracetamol, eight out of 10 who received N-acetyl cysteine within 10 hours of paracetamol ingestion delivered normal infants (the remaining two opted for therapeutic abortion). However, only five out of 10 who received N-acetyl cysteine within 10–16 hours of paracetamol ingestion delivered normal infants (two opted for therapeutic abortion and three aborted spontaneously). Whilst of the four patients who did not receive N-acetyl cysteine until 16 hours after ingestion of paracetamol, one died and the remaining three all aborted spontaneously. Obviously, paracetamol should be avoided in babies with jaundice.

NSAIDs

Although non steroidal anti-inflammatory drugs (NSAIDs) have been shown to be effective analgesic agents in older children there is very little efficacy and safety data for infants, and none of the NSAIDs is currently licensed for analgesic use in infants under six months of age. In the UK, diclofenac and ibuprofen are not licensed for use in children of less than one year. The pharmacokinetics of NSAIDs are probably similar in infants aged over three months to those in adults.[44] In preterm neonates the plasma elimination half-life of intravenous indomethacin (given to promote closure of patent ductus arteriosus) is three times longer than in adults and clearance is three times lower, possibly due to immature renal function and hepatic metabolism.[45] Aspirin, with its anti-inflammatory properties, has in the past been widely used as an analgesic agent in children. Neonates eliminate aspirin more slowly than adults but the elimination half-life reaches adult levels within the first year of life. However, the association between the use of aspirin and the development of Reye's Syndrome, has resulted in a recommendation by the UK Committee on the Safety of Medicines that aspirin should not be given to children under 12 years of age, either for analgesia or as an antipyretic.

Opioid analgesic drugs

Morphine

Opioid pharmacology is now better understood in children and, as in adults, morphine remains the standard opioid for the treatment of pain. However, there is a declining enthusiasm for intramuscular opioid injections, which result in fluctuating plasma drug levels and cycles of pain, comfort and sedation.[46]

In a retrospective survey of 933 neonates following major surgery Purcell Jones and colleagues[47] found that 131 patients (14%) had received an opioid as part of their anaesthetic. Two hundred and forty patients were electively ventilated postoperatively and of these 88 had received an opioid. A further 51 patients who had received an opioid were allowed to breathe spontaneously postoperatively. These authors concluded that the safest opioids for use with spontaneous respiration were codeine phosphate (in a dose of 1 mg/kg intramuscularly) and morphine (in a dose of 0.1 mg/kg intramuscularly). Intravenous infusion of morphine 10 µg/kg/h was also considered safe.

Neonates and infants of less than six months are particularly susceptible to the respiratory depressant effects of opioids.[48] There are a number of reasons for the sensitivity of neonates to opioids including: altered pharmacokinetics;[49] increased permeability of the blood-brain barrier;[50] increased amounts of endogenous opioids and developmental changes in the opioid receptor population.[51] The elimination half-life of morphine in neonates is five times longer than in adults; the clearance of morphine in neonates is only one-fortieth of that in adults but the volume of distribution of the drug is much the same in neonates and adults. Even greater differences exist in pre-term neonates (Table 8.2).[49,52–54] Hence the need for lower infusion rates in infants than older children. Morphine is metabolized to morphine-6–glucuronide, which is active; morphine-3-glucuronide, which is inactive, and also morphine sulphate. Glucuronidation is impaired in the neonatal period.[52]

All intravenous techniques demand continuous direct supervision by specially trained staff, but this should not restrict their use to an intensive care setting. In addition, apnoea monitors should be used whenever opioids are administered to infants less than 6 months of age. In order to mini-

Table 8.2 Morphine pharmacokinetics in neonates and adults[49,52–54]

	Half-life (h)	Clearance (ml/min/kg)
Neonates of 26–30 weeks	6–14	3.4
Term babies	2–11	4.7–6.3
Adults	2.9	11.5–15

mize the risk of errors simple dilution and infusion rates based on body weight should be used (Table 8.3).[48] A loading dose of 100–200 µg/kg morphine may be given before commencing the infusion. A simple continuous morphine infusion usually provides satisfactory analgesia, but, depending on circumstances, analgesic requirements vary widely between patients and in the same patient. Altering the infusion rate of morphine within the limits defined in Table 8.3 will only slowly alter plasma concentration and clinical effect. Analgesic requirements can more easily be tailored to the individual child's requirements using PCA.

Table 8.3   Administration of morphine by infusion (adapted from reference 48, with permission)

Dose of morphine	Dilution	Concentration	Infusion rate
0.5 mg/kg body weight	Make up to 50 ml with 5% dextrose	1 ml/h = 10 µg/kg/h	*Neonates* 0.5–1.5 ml/h 5–15 µg/kg/h *Older children* 0.5–4.0 ml/h 5–40 µg/kg/h

PCA has been used succesfully in children as young as five years of age. Berde and colleagues[46] studied children following major orthopaedic surgery, and found that patients receiving either PCA alone or PCA with a background infusion had lower pain scores and greater satisfaction than patients receiving intramuscularly administered morphine. Unfortunately it is a common observation that bolus-only PCA in children results in poor pain relief and sedation. The addition of a background infusion might be expected to result in superior analgesia. The study by Berde and colleagues[46] found that the addition of a background infusion of morphine (15 µg/kg/h) to PCA resulted in an improvement in analgesia without any increase in side effects. Gaukroger and colleagues[55] used a very similar background infusion rate of morphine (16 µg/kg/h) also without adverse effect. Several studies have found that background infusions increase the incidence of side effects without improving analgesia. Doyle and colleagues[56] found that a background infusion of morphine (20 µg/kg/h) did not improve pain scores although it was associated with a better sleep pattern. However, this infusion rate was also associated with a greater incidence of hypoxaemia, excessive sedation, nausea and vomiting compared with a PCA-only regimen. Interestingly, Doyle and colleagues[57] have shown in a subsequent study that PCA, in combination with a very low dose background infusion rate of morphine (4 µg/kg/h), is associated with a better sleep pattern, less hypoxia and less nausea and vomiting than PCA with either no background infusion or with a background infusion rate of 10 µg/kg/min. The rationale for this effect remains obscure.

Codeine

Codeine phosphate is an effective opioid analgesic in neonates and infants. The half-life of codeine in postoperative infants is similar to that in adults[58] but there is no data on the pharmacokinetics of codeine in neonates. Codeine is metabolized to norcodeine, codeine-6–phosphate and morphine, all of which have analgesic activity. A single dose of 1 mg/kg is often all that is required, following which the risk of respiratory depression is minimal. However, respiratory depression can occur following multiple doses[47] particularly in the younger age group. These patients should be closely monitored. Codeine phosphate may be administered orally or by intramuscular injection, but should never be given intravenously as this can cause apnoea and severe hypotension.[59]

Fentanyl

The potency and lack of sedative or hypnotic properties have not made fentanyl popular for conventional postoperative analgesia in the UK. Fentanyl has a high clearance with a very variable plasma half-life in neonates.[60] It is particularly influenced by the decrease in liver blood flow which occur with most inhalational anaesthetics. Nevertheless, Chambers and colleagues[61] have found that intravenous fentanyl (1–2 μg/kg) provides acceptable postoperative analgesia following circumcision. Fentanyl provides excellent analgesia when administered as a patient-controlled epidural infusion (PCEA) but may be associated with increased sedation particularly when infused in the thoracic region.[62]

Pethidine

In children, pethidine is used for premedication more commonly than for postoperative pain management and there would seem to be little benefit in using pethidine in preference to morphine postoperatively. Indeed, repeat dosing with pethidine in adults can cause seizures due to the accumulation of norpethidine. A recent study was unable to recommend the rectal route of administration of pethidine in children, as it was associated with wide variations in bioavailability.[63]

Regional analgesia and nerve blocks

Pharmacokinetics of local anaesthetic agents

Ralston and Shnider[64] have reviewed the effects of regional anaesthesia in neonates following delivery and report that, as in adults, local anaesthetic metabolism is oxidative. However, there are variable changes in drug half-life; that of bupivacaine is unchanged but that of lignocaine is prolonged.

In infants, peak plasma concentrations of bupivacaine following caudal block may occur as early as 10 minutes after block placement compared with 30 minutes in adults. However, the elimination half-life is considerably longer in children than adults. Mazoit and colleagues[65] investigated the pharmacokinetics of caudal 0.5% bupivacaine (2.5 mg/kg) in infants aged from one to six months. The half-life in this age group (7.5 hours) was some two to three times longer than in adults. Bupivacaine binds to alpha-1–acid glycoprotein and albumin. However, the free fraction of bupivacaine, although decreasing with increasing age, was dangerously high in a few patients in this study. In contrast, Eyres and colleagues[66] found that plasma concentrations following caudal 0.25% bupivacaine (3 mg/kg) in 45 children whose ages ranged from 4 months to 12 years were 1.2 to 1.4 µg/ml (i.e. well below toxic levels). Bricker and colleagues[67] investigated the pharmacokinetics of intercostal 0.25% bupivacaine (1.5 mg/kg) in 11 neonates under 3 kg. The peak concentration of 0.82 µg/ml occurred within 10 minutes and the half-life was 132 minutes. Similar results were obtained in 11 older infants. Plasma bupivacaine levels following ilio-inguinal combined with ilio-hypogastric nerve block for orchidopexy were similarly well below toxic levels.[68]

Extradural spinal anaesthesia

The shorter, straighter spine of neonates and the fact that the extradural space is less densely packed with fat will permit a catheter to be fed from the sacrococcygeal ligament to the thoracic or lumbar region. In older children catheters are inserted at the required level. Epidural local anaesthetic agents provide excellent analgesia with few systemic side effects, and the hypotension that occurs in adults is rare in children.[69] As experience with paediatric epidurals increases it has become evident that there is a high incidence of technical problems involving needles and catheters.[70] In a series of 174 children, infusion of local anaesthetic via indwelling pleural and epidural catheters was found to provide safe, effective analgesia and eliminated the need for systemic opioids in the majority of children.[71] This series compared the results of epidural catheters placed in the thoracic, lumbar and caudal spaces. Thoracic and lumbar catheter placement was difficult. However, caudal epidural insertion with the catheter passed up to the thoracic region, although easier, was associated with the highest frequency of supplemental medication requirement and a high (22%) failure rate. Patients who have received extradural opioids must be appropriately observed for 24 hours following their cessation.[72]

Wolf and Hughes[73] compared epidural 0.25% bupivacaine (0.1–0.15 ml/kg/h) with intravenous morphine and found both to be equally effective for analgesia in infants undergoing abdominal surgery. Patients in the intravenous morphine group were significantly more sedated. Conversely, in the extradural group, lack of sedation was troublesome in some infants over

6 months. Although peripheral oxygen saturation was reduced in the intravenous morphine group, this was not of clinical significance.

Problems with inadequate sedation during extradural infusion of local anaesthetic have been previously reported but not in infants or neonates under three months.[74] It is important not to interpret the lack of sedation as inadequate analgesia and increase the extradural infusion rate, as this can lead to local anaesthetic toxicity. Berde has constructed a set of guidelines to avoid this eventuality.[75] If opioids are infused together with local anaesthetics in the extradural space, sedation is improved but the incidence of complications rises. Pruritus occurs in 10–40% of children, nausea and vomiting in 10–40%, and up to 50% develop retention of urine, this latter complication being more common in older children.[62,76] Wilson and Lloyd-Thomas[74] have reviewed the safety of extradural infusions using a diamorphine-bupivacaine mixture. With close observation of the patient, paying particular attention to the level of sedation, the technique was felt to be safe. Fentanyl is particularly suitable for epidural administration. Candle and colleagues have reported encouraging results using PCA for the administration of fentanyl.[62]

Two feared, but fortunately rare, complications of paediatric extradural analgesia are convulsions from local anaesthetic toxicity and respiratory depression from opioid overdose.[77,78] A collaborative study involving 15 paediatric centres worldwide analysed the factors associated with these two adverse events among over 40 000 paediatric regional anaesthetics.[79] In the main these two complications were associated with excessive dosing and can be made very rare by limiting the bupivacaine dose to 0.4 to 0.5 mg/kg/h, and by limiting epidural morphine boluses in opioid-naive patients to 0.05 mg/kg, or by limiting epidural morphine infusion to 5 μg/kg/h. Other, less severe complications of continuous epidural infusions of bupivacaine were retrospectively studied in 190 patients.[80] In order of frequency the complications were nausea and vomiting (23%), excessive motor blockade (15.8%), oversedation (6.3%) and pruritus (5.2%).

Caudal anaesthesia

Caudal block is one of the most common local anaesthetic techniques in children, being used to supplement general anaesthesia for a wide variety of 'sacral segment' surgery. Caudal anaesthesia has even been used as the sole anaesthetic for inguinal herniotomy in awake ex-premature neonates.[81]

It would seem that larger volumes of more dilute solutions of local anaesthetic should be preferred.[82,83] Wolf and colleagues[82] demonstrated that caudal 0.125% bupivacaine provided analgesia that lasted as long as more concentrated solutions. Broadman and colleagues[83] have gone so far as to say that there is no advantage to be gained by increasing the concentration of bupivacaine above 0.25%. These same authors investigated the complications of caudals, both short term and long term, in a very large series.

Caudal block placement using 0.25% bupivacaine (3 mg/kg) was performed in 1154 consecutive cases of children whose ages ranged from 1 month to 18 years. Sixty five per cent of blocks were performed on ambulatory surgery patients with no long term complications.[84] Many anaesthetists perform caudal block placement before surgery. However, Holthusen and colleagues[85] have found that there is no pre-emptive analgesic advantage gained by performing caudal block placement before compared with after surgery.

Caudal analgesia with opioids is not recommended for outpatient surgery because of a high incidence of urinary retention and an uncommon but real chance of delayed respiratory depression. 'Single shot' caudal morphine, 0.03 µg/kg for lower dermatomes and 0.05 µg/kg for thoracic dermatome block, provides more prolonged analgesia than local anaesthetic alone and is effective for thoracic as well as lumbosacral dermatomes.[86,87] A recent retrospective analysis of 138 children who had received caudal morphine included 42 children younger than 6 months of age and 15 less than 1 month of age.[88] The incidence of clinically important respiratory depression in this series was 8%, higher than in any equivalent adult series. Furthermore, 10 of the 11 cases occurred in children under one year of age and weighing less than 9 kg. Caudal buprenorphine has been reported to be equally as effective as caudal morphine.[89]

Subarachnoid spinal anaesthesia

One of the earliest reports of the use of spinal anaesthesia for surgery in infants and children was presented by Tyrrell-Gray in 1910.[90] In this series of 300 spinal anaesthetics there was one death in a gravely ill child. Despite this, spinals have been recommended as the anaesthetic of choice in high-risk neonates.[91] Two recent studies have assessed the haemodynamic effects of subarachnoid block.[92,93] In infants less than 6 months old spinal bupivacaine (0.3 mg/kg) was associated with haemodynamic instability [92] whereas in preterm infants the technique was not associated with haemodynamic instability.[93] Awake regional anaesthetic techniques in neonates often require supplemental sedation intraoperatively and this increases complications. Welborn and colleagues reported a very high incidence (89%) of apnoea in infants who received spinal anaesthesia supplemented by ketamine sedation.[94]

Intercostal block

In a study of 14 children (age range 2 months to 17 years), following thoracotomy Tobias and colleagues[95] concluded that interpleural catheter placement for infusion of local anaesthetic provided effective analgesia with no complications.

Ilio-inguinal and ilio-hypogastric block

The combination of ilio-inguinal and ilio-hypogastric nerve block can provide effective analgesia for orchidopexy[96] and hernia repair.[68] In a study of 44 boys undergoing ambulatory surgery, children who had ilio-inguinal and ilio-hypogastric nerve block reported similar analgesia to caudal block.[96] These authors, like Chambers and colleagues,[61] reported that intravenous fentanyl (1–2 µg/kg) provided acceptable 'rescue' analgesia.

Penile block

Penile block is a safe, simple, effective method for analgesia in circumcision, especially in children. Penile block provides good intraoperative and postoperative analgesia but the technique requires skill and in particular may cause haematomas. Injection of local anaesthetic on each side is more reliable than a single mid-line injection under the symphysis pubis.[61,97] However, a study in adult circumcisions by Serour and colleagues[98] suggests that the perineal branch of the pudendal nerve (which supplies the ventral aspect of the penis), should also be anaesthetised during penile block. An alternative is simply to inject a subcutaneous ring of bupivacaine around the base of the penis shaft.[99]

Instillation of local anaesthetic

Subcutaneous infiltration of the skin and underlying tissues, to block nerve conduction at the most terminal branches of the sensory nerves, is a commonly used technique in paediatric surgical practice. Simple instillation of local anaesthetic in the open wound was found to be equally as effective as ilio-inguinal and ilio-hypogastric nerve block after inguinal hernia repair.[100] In contrast Conroy and colleagues[101] found that wound instillation was inferior to caudal block with respect to pain-related behaviour in children following inguinal herniorrhaphy. Topical lignocaine jelly (applied on completion of surgery[61] and EMLA cream[102] are both less effective than dorsal nerve block of the penis for post-circumcision analgesia.

Other drugs

Clonidine

Several studies have demonstrated that clonidine added to the local anaesthetic in epidural[103,104] and caudal blocks[105,106] both enhances and prolongs the analgesia produced by the block. A dose of clonidine (3 µg/kg) epidurally[103] and up to 5 µg/kg caudally[105,106] is not associated with any significant haemodynamic or sedative effect but 5 µg/kg epidurally is associated with lower blood pressure and heart rate postoperatively.[104]

KEY POINTS FOR CLINICAL PRACTICE

- Nociception is associated with symptoms and signs of distress even in newborn infants. Untreated pain in neonates is associated with excess morbidity and mortality.
- Assessment of pain in children is necessary to assist effective analgesic therapy. However, assessment may be difficult, particularly in the pre-verbal in child. Behavioural measures commonly assess fear and anxiety as well as pain. Self-reporting measures may be reliable in older children.
- Paracetamol can be used safely in nearly all children, including neonates who would appear to be resistant to the toxic effects of paracetamol.
- Opioids with a high therapeutic margin can be used safely in children older than 6 months. Care and close monitoring are essential if opioids are to be used in children under 6 months.
- Regional blockade for peri-operative pain relief is associated with excellent results. However, pain may be troublesome once the block has worn off so adjuvant analgesic therapy is essential.

REFERENCES

1. Rogers M. Do the right thing – pain relief in infants and children (editorial). N Eng J Med 1992; 326: 55–56
2. International Association for the Study of Pain. Pain terms: a list with definitions and notes on usage. Pain 1979; 6: 249–251
3. The Royal College of Surgeons of England and College of Anaesthetists. Commission on the Provision of Surgical Services. Report of the Working Party on Pain after Surgery. Her Majesty's Stationery Office, London, 1990
4. Choonara I A. Pain relief. Arch Disease Child 1989; 64: 1101–1102
5. Audit Commission. Children First. Her Majesty's Stationery Office, London, 1993
6. Anonymous. Treating moderate and severe pain in infants. Drug Ther Bull 1984; 32 (3): 21–24
7. Yaster M. Analgesia and anesthesia in neonates (editorial). J Pediatr 1987; 111: 394–396
8. McCaffery M, Hart L. Undertreatment of acute pain with narcotics. Am J Nurs 1976; 76: 1586–1591
9. Beyer J E, DeGood D E, Ashley L C, Russel G A. Patterns of post-operative analgesic use with adults and children following cardiac surgery. Pain 1983; 17: 71–81
10. Mather L, Mackie J. The incidence of post-operative pain in children. Pain 1983; 15: 271–282
11. Sriwatankul K, Weis O F, Alloza J L, Kelvie W, Weintraub M. Analysis of narcotic analgesic usage in the treatment of post-operative pain. JAMA 1983; 250: 926–929
12. Schechter N L, Allen D A, Hanson K. Status of paediatric pain control: A comparison of hospital analgesic usage in children and adults. Paediatrics 1986; 77: 11–15
13. Rana SR. Pain – A subject ignored. Paediatrics 1987; 79: 309
14. Choonara I. Management of pain in newborn infants. Seminars in Perinatology 1992; 16: 32–40
15. Anand K J S, Hickey P R. Pain and its effects in the human neonate and fetus. N Engl J Med 1987; 317: 1321–1329
16. Anand K J S, Hickey P R. Halothane-morphine compared with high dose sufentanil for anesthesia and post-operative analgesia in neonatal cardiac surgery. N Engl J Med 1992; 326: 1–9

17. Craig K D, Whitfield M F, Grunau R V E, Linton J, Hadjistavropoulos H D. Pain in the preterm neonate: behavioural and physiological indices. Pain 1993; 52: 287–299
18. Porter F. Pain assessment in children: infants. In: Schechter N L, Berde C B, Yaster M (eds) Pain in Infants, Children and Adolescents. Williams and Wilkins, Baltimore, 1993; pp 87–96
19. Fitzgerald M, McIntosh N. Pain and analgesia in the newborn. Arch Dis Child 1989; 64: 441–443
20. Charnay Y, Paulin C, Dray F et al. Distribution of enkephalin in human fetus and infant spinal cord: an immunofluorescence study. J Comp Neurol 1984; 223: 415–423
21. Fitzgerald M. Development of pain mechanisms. Br Med Bull 1991; 47: 667–675
22. Besson J M, Chaouch A. Peripheral and spinal mechanisms of nociception. Physiol Reviews 1987; 67: 67–186
23. Woolf C J. Recent advances in the pathophysiology of acute pain. Br J Anaesth 1989; 63: 139–146
24. Beyer J E, McGrath P J, Berde C B. Discordance between self report and behavioural pain measures in children aged 3–7 years after surgery. J Pain Sympt Mana 1990; 5: 350–356
25. Craig K D, McMahon R J, Morrison J D, Zaskow C. Developmental changes in infant pain expression during immunisation injections. Social Science and Medicine 1984; 19: 1331–1337
26. Robieux I, Kumar R, Radhakrishan S, Koren G. Assessing pain and analgesia with a lidocaine-prilocaine emulsion in infants and toddlers during venipuncture. J Pediatr 1991: 118; 971–973
27. Jacqz-Aigrain E, Dauod P, Burtin P et al. Placebo-controlled trial of midazolam sedation in mechanically ventilated newborn babies. Lancet 1994: 344; 646–648
28. Katz E R, Kellerman J, Siegal S E. Behavioural distress in children with cancer undergoing medical procedures: developmental considerations. J Consult Clin Psychol 1980: 48; 356–365
29. Katz E R, Kellerman J, Siegal S E. Anxiety as an effective focus in the clinical study of acute behavioural distress. J Consulting Clin Psychol 1981: 49; 470–471
30. McGrath P J, Johnson G, Goodman J et al. The CHEOPS: a behavioural scale to measure post-operative pain in children. In: Fields H L, Dubner R, Cervero F (eds) Advances in Pain Research and Therapy. Raven Press, New York, 1985
31. McGrath P A, de Veber L L, Hearn M T. Multidimensional pain assessment in children. Adv Pain Res Ther 1985: 9; 387–393
32. Hester N O. The preoperational child's reaction to immunisation. Nurs Res 1979: 28; 250–254
33. Eland J M, Anderson J E. The experience of pain in children. In: Jacox A K (ed). Pain: a source book for nurses and other health professionals. Little Brown, Boston, 1977
34. Franck L S. A national survey of the assessment and treatment of pain and agitation in the neonatal intensive care unit. J Obstet Gynecol Neonat Nurs 1987; 16: 387–393
35. Miller R P, Roberts R J, Fisher L J. Acetaminophen elimination kinetics in neonates, children and adults. Clin Pharmacol Ther 1976; 19: 284–294
36. Hopkins C S, Underhill S, Booker P D. Pharmacokinetics of paracetamol after cardiac surgery. Arch Dis Child 1990; 65: 971–976.
37. Gaudreault P, Nicol O, Dupuis C. Pharmacokinetics and clinical efficacy of intrarectal solution of acetaminophen. Can J Anaesth 1988; 35: 149–152
38. Depre M, van Hecken A, Verbesselt R et al. Tolerance of propacetamol, a paracetamol formulation for intravenous use. Fundamentals Clin Pharmacol 1992; 6: 259–262
39. Granry J C, Rod B, Boccard E et al. Pharmacokinetics and antipyretic effects of an injectable pro-drug of paracetamol (propacetamol) in children. Paed Anaesth 1992; 2: 291–295
40. Peterson R G, Rumack B G. Pharmacokinetics of acetaminophen in children. Paediatrics 1978; 62: 877–879
41. Notorianni L J, Oldham H G, Bennett P N. Passage of paracetamol into breast

milk and its subsequent metabolism by the neonate. Br J Clin Pharmacol 1987; 24: 63–67

42. Lieh-Lai M W, Sarnaik A P, Newton J F. Metabolism and pharmacokinetics of acetaminophen in a severely poisoned young child. J Pediatr 1984; 105: 125–128

43. Riggs B S, Bronstein A C, Kulig K et al. Acute acetamiophen overdose during pregnancy. Obstet Gynecol 1989; 74: 247–253

44. Kauffman R E , Nelson M V. Effect of age on ibuprofen pharmacokinetics and antipyretic response. J Pediatr 1992; 121: 969–973

45. Thalji A A, Carr I, Yeh T F et al. Pharmacokinetics of intravenously administered indomethacin in preterm infants. J Pediatr 1980; 97: 995–1000

46. Berde C B, Lehn B M Yee J D et al. Patient controlled analgesia in children and adolescents: A randomized, prospective comparison with intramuscular administration of morphine for post-operative analgesia. J Pediatr 1991; 118: 460–466

47. Purcell-Jones G, Dormon F, Sumner E. The use of opioids in neonates, a retrospective study of 933 cases. Anaesthesia 1987; 42: 1316–1320

48. Lloyd-Thomas D. Pain management in paediatric patients. Br J Anaesth 1990; 64: 85–104

49. Choonara I, Laurence A, Michalkiewicz A et al. Morphine metabolism in neonates and infants. Br J Clin Pharmacol 1992; 34: 434–437

50. Kupferburg H J, Way E L. Pharmacological basis for the increased sensitivity of the newborn rat to morphine. J Pharmacol Exp Ther 1963; 141: 105–112

51. Lesley R M, Tso S, Holbutt T E. Differential appearance of opiate receptor subtypes in neonatal rat brain. Life Sci 1982; 31: 1393–1396

52. Lynn A M, Slattery J T. Morphine pharmacokinetics in early pregnancy. Anesthesiology 1987; 66: 136–139

53. Choonara I A, McKay P, Hain R et al. Morphine metabolism in children. Br J Clin Pharmacol 1989; 28: 599–604

54. Bhat R, Chari C, Gulati A et al. Pharmacokinetics of a single dose of morphine in pre-term infants during the first week of life. J Pediatr 1990; 117: 477–481

55. Gaukroger P B, Tomkins D P, van der Walt J H. Patient controlled analgesia in children. Anaesth Intens Care 1989; 17: 264–268

56. Doyle E, Robinson D, Morton NS. Comparison of PCA with and without a background infusion after lower abdominal surgery in children. Br J Anaesth 1993; 71: 670–673

57. Doyle E, Harper I, Morton N S. PCA with low dose background infusions after lower abdominal surgery in children. Br J Anaesth 1993; 71: 818–822

58. Olsson G L, Quiding H, Boreus L-O et al. Pharmacokinetics of codeine in postoperative paediatric patients. Pain 1990 suppl 5: S7

59. Yaster M, Deshpande J K. Management of pediatric pain with opioid analgesics. J Pediatr 1988: 113; 421–429

60. Koehntop D E, Rodman J H, Brundge D M et al. Pharmacokinetics of fentanyl in neonates. Anesth Analg 1986; 65: 227–232

61. Chambers F A, Lee J, Smith J, Casey W. Post circumcision analgesia: a comparison of topical analgesia with dorsal nerve block using the midline and lateral approaches. Br J Anaesth 1994; 73: 437–439

62. Candle C L, Freid E B, Bailey A G et al. Epidural fentanyl infusion with patient-controlled epidural analgesia for postoperative analgesia in children. J Pediatr Surg 1993; 28: 554–559

63. Hamunen K, Maunuksela E-L, Seppala T, Olkkola K T. Pharmacokinetics of I.V. and rectal pethidine in children undergoing ophthalmic surgery. Br J Anaesth 1993; 71: 823–826

64. Ralston D H, Shnider S M. The fetal and neonatal effects of regional anesthesia in obstetrics. Anesthesiology 1978; 48: 34–64

65. Mazoit J X, Denson D D, Samii K. Pharmacokinetics of bupivacaine following caudal anesthesia in infants. Anesthesiology 1988; 68: 387–391

66. Eyres R L, Bishop W, Oppenheim R C, Brown T C K. Plasma bupivacaine concentrations in children during caudal epidural analgesia. Anaesth Intens Care 1983; 11: 20–22

67. Bricker S R, Telford R J, Booker P D. Pharmacokinetics of bupivacaine following

intraoperative intercostal nerve block in neonates and infants aged less than 6 months. Anesthesiology 1989; 70: 942–947

68. Epstein R H, Larijani G E, Wolfson P J et al. Plasma bupivacaine concentrations following ilioinguinal-iliohypogastric nerve blockade in children. Anesthesiology 1988; 69: 773–776

69. Dalens B, Chrysostome Y. Intervertebral epidural anaesthesia in paediatric surgery: success rate and adverse effects in 650 consecutive procedures. Paed Anaesth 1991: 1; 107–117

70. Wood C E, Goresky G V, Klassen K A et al. Complications of continuous epidural infusions for post-operative analgesia in children. Can J Anaesth 1994: 41; 613–620

71. Pietropaoli J A Jnr, Keller M S, Small D F et al. Regional anesthesia in pediatric surgery: complications and postoperative comfort level in 174 consecutive children. J Pediatr Surg 1993: 28: 560–564

72. Nicholls D G, Yaster M, Lynn A M et al. Disposition and respiratory effects of intrathecal morphine in children. Anesthesiology 1993: 79; 733–738

73. Wolf A R, Hughes D. Pain relief for infants undergoing abdominal surgery: comparison of infusions of IV morphine and extradural bupivacaine. Br J Anaesth 1993: 70; 10–16

74. Wilson P T J, Lloyd-Thomas A R. An audit of extradural infusion analgesia in children using bupivacaine and diamorphine. Anaesthesia 1993: 48; 718–723

75. Berde C B. Convulsions associated with pediatric regional analgesia. Anesth Analg 1992: 75; 164–166

76. Lloyd-Thomas A R, Howard R. A pain service for children. Pediatr Anaesth 1994: 4; 3–15

77. McCloskey J J, Haun S E , Deshpande J K. Bupivacaine toxicity secondary to continuous caudal epidural infusion in children. Anesth Analg 1992: 75; 287–290

78. Agarwal R, Gutlove D P, Lockhart C H. Seizures occurring in pediatric patients receiving continuous infusion of bupivacaine. Anesth Analg 1992: 75; 284–286

79. Berde C. Epidural analgesia in children (editorial). Can J Anaesth 1994; 41: 555–560

80. Wood C E, Goresky G V, Klassen K A, Nail S. Complications of continuous epidural infusions for post-operative analgesia in children. Can J Anaesth 1994; 41: 613–620

81. Peutrell J M, Hughes D G. Epidural anaesthesia through caudal catheters for inguinal herniotomies in awake ex-premature babies. Anaesthesia 1993; 48: 128–131

82. Wolf A R, Valley R, Fear D W et al. Bupivacaine for caudal analgesia in infants and children: the optimal effective concentration. Anesthesiology 1988; 69: 102–106

83. Broadman L M, Hannallah R S, Norie W C et al. Caudal analgesia in pediatric outpatient surgery: a comparison of three different bupivacaine concentrations. Anesth Analg 1987; 66 (suppl): S19

84. Broadman L M, Hannallah R S, Norden J M, McGill W A. 'Kiddie Caudals' experience with 1154 consecutive cases without complications. Anesth Analg 1987; 66 (suppl): S18

85. Holthusen H, Eichwede F, Stevens M et al. Pre-emptive analgesia: a comparison of preoperative with postoperative caudal block on postoperative pain in children. Br J Anaesth 1994; 73: 440–442

86. Krane E J, Jacobson L E, Lynn A M et al. Caudal morphine for post-operative analgesia in children: a comparison with caudal bupivacaine and intravenous morphine. Anesth Analg 1987; 66: 647–653

87. Krane E J, Tyler D C, Jacobson L E. The dose response of caudal morphine in children. Anesthesiology 1989; 71: 48–52

88. Valley R D, Bailey A G. Caudal morphine for postoperative analgesia in infants and children: a report of 138 cases. Anesth Analg 1991; 72: 120–124

89. Girotra S, Kumar S, Rajendran K M. Comparison of caudal morphine and buprenorphine for post-operative analgesia in children. Eur J Anaesth 1993; 10: 309–312

90. Tyrrell-Gray H. A further study of spinal anaesthesia in children and infants. Lancet 1910: (11 June) 1611–1616

91. Abajian J C, Mellish P W, Browne A E et al. Spinal anesthesia for surgery in the high-risk infant. Anesth Analg 1984; 63: 359–362
92. Mahe V, Ecoffey C. Spinal anesthesia with isobaric bupivacaine in infants. Anesthesiology 1988; 68: 601–603
93. Gallagher T M, Crean P M. Spinal anaesthesia in infants born prematurely. Anaesthesia 1989; 44: 434–436
94. Welborn L G, Rice I J, Hannallah R S et al. Postoperative apnoea in former preterm infants: prospective comparison of spinal and general anesthesia. Anesthesiology 1990; 72: 838–842
95. Tobias J D, Martin L D, Oakes L et al. Postoperative analgesia following thoracotomy in children: interpleural catheters. J Pediatr Surg 1993; 28: 1466–1470
96. Hannallah R S, Broadman L M, Belman A B et al. Comparison of caudal and ilioinguinal/iliohypogastric nerve blocks for control of post-orchidopexy pain in pediatric ambulatory surgery. Anesthesiology 1987; 66: 832–834
97. Brown T C K, Weidner N J, Bouwmeester J. Dorsal nerve of penis block: anatomical and radiological studies. Anaesth Intens Care 1989; 17: 34–38
98. Serour F, Mori J, Barr J. Optimal regional anesthesia for circumcision. Anesth Analg 1994; 79: 129–131
99. Broadman L M, Hannallah R S, Belman A B et al. Post circumcision pain – a prospective evaluation of subcutaneous ring block of the penis. Anesthesiology 1987; 67: 399–402
100. Casey W F, Rice R S, Broadman L et al. A comparison between bupivacaine instillation versus ilioinguinal/iliohypogastric nerve block for postoperative analgesia following inguinal herniorrhaphy. Anesthesiology 1990; 72: 637–639
101. Conroy J M, Othersen H B Jnr, Dorman B H et al. A comparison of wound instillation and caudal block for analgesia following pediatric inguinal herniorrhaphy. J Pediatr Surg 1993; 28: 565–567
102. Lee J J, Forrester P. EMLA for postoperative analgesia for day case circumcision in children. A comparison with dorsal nerve penis block. Anaesthesia 1992; 47: 1081–1083
103. Rochette A, Beauvar M D, Raux O et al. Clonidine prolongation of epidural blockade in children. Anesthesiology 1994; 81: A1340
104. Motsch M D, Bach A, Bohrer H et al. Addition of clonidine enhances and prolongs postoperative analgesia from caudal bupivacaine in children. Anesthesiology 1993; 79: A1138
105. Beauvar C, Rochette A, Raux O et al. Clonidine prolongation of caudal anesthetic in children. Anesthesiology 1994; 81: A1347
106. Klimscha W, Sanberer A, Lerche A et al. Caudal block with clonidine provides prolonged analgesia after ambulatory hernia repair in children. Anesthesiology 1994; 81: A952

9

Non-acute pain

D. Justins

In 1993 The Royal College of Anaesthetists, The Association of Anaesthetists and The Pain Society published 'Anaesthetists and Non-acute Pain' which addressed the provision and organization of pain management services in the UK. Guidelines were also given for training in non-acute pain relief, a neglected subject. Health purchasers and policy making bodies are beginning to listen and the provision of services for non-acute pain has received high priority in some places.

WHAT IS NON-ACUTE PAIN?

The term non-acute pain encompasses pains variously described as chronic, persistent or intractable. Chronic pain has been defined as pain which persists past the time when healing is expected to be complete but this definition is inadequate. In some cases of chronic pain, for example rheumatoid arthritis, there may be ongoing tissue damage so that healing is never complete. In other cases there has never been any evidence of tissue damage which needs to heal nor any other likely pathophysiological cause. Psychological factors may be important in such cases.[1]

HOW COMMON IS NON-ACUTE PAIN?

It has proved very difficult to determine the real incidence of non-acute pain in the community. A telephone survey in the UK[2] reported that 11% of people contacted said that they suffered from chronic pain and that a further 8% said that someone else in their household suffered from chronic pain. Back and neck pain represent the largest group in most surveys; back pain is cited as the cause of over 45 million certified days off work in Britain every year. The casemix seen in pain clinics may not be representative of the general patient population, let alone the general community. Data from one pain clinic revealed that low back pain (26%), postherpetic neuralgia (11%) and post-traumatic neuralgia (9%) were the commonest conditions.[3] As pain management in primary care improves then we may see only intractable cases in the pain clinic.

ECONOMICS

Bonica estimated that in 1983 some 90 million Americans suffered chronic pain at a cost of $US 70 billion.[4] In the UK the annual cost of back pain to the National Health Service has been estimated at approximately £480 million.[5] A survey of patients attending a pain clinic in New Zealand revealed that on average these patients visited their general practitioners 12.9 times per year compared with 4.2 times per year for the general population.[6] Because of the underprovision of pain relief services the resulting delay before seeing a pain specialist may prevent treatment being given at the optimal time and prejudice recovery.[7]

THE PATHOPHYSIOLOGY OF NON-ACUTE PAIN

Nociceptive pain results from ongoing activation of physiologically normal nerve fibres which may be somatic (e.g. tumour invasion, arthritis) or visceral (e.g. ureteric colic, hepatomegaly). Neurogenic or neuropathic pain is associated with abnormality, injury or disease in the nervous system. This includes painful mononeuropathies (e.g. intercostal neuralgia), polyneuropathies (e.g. diabetes mellitus), deafferentation pain (e.g. brachial plexus avulsion, central post stroke pain) and sympathetically maintained pain (SMP). SMP may or may not be associated with nerve injury. There is a group of patients in whom the symptom of pain may be predominately due to, or associated with, psychological factors. A patient with non-acute pain may have components of nociceptive, neurogenic and psychological pain.

The gate control theory, published in 1965, only hinted at the complex neurophysiology of nociception.[8] The transduction of a peripheral nociceptive stimulus into the consciously perceived experience of pain involves a complex, plastic system which uses a large number of excitatory, facilitatory, and inhibitory neurotransmitters and receptor types. Even a brief peripheral nociceptive stimulus is capable of inducing long lasting changes in the functional configuration of the dorsal horn. Nociceptive neurones in the dorsal horn may discharge in the absence of any peripheral drive. Peripherally acting drugs or interruption of the peripheral pathways are often ineffective.[9] Visceral pain involves separate mechanisms.

The attention of researchers has been focused on the inhibitory component of pain modulation but there are now suggestions that the facilitatory component may play an important role in some pain states.[10] This is further evidence that sensory drive from peripheral primary afferent nociceptor neurones may not be required to drive nociceptive neurones in the dorsal horn or central nervous system.

There is also a resurgence of interest in the brain. It is unlikely that complex non-acute pain problems will be explained purely on the basis of peripheral noxious stimuli and resulting neurochemical events. The move back towards the brain allows us to consider pain in a broad biopsychosocial context rather than in a purely traditional stimulus-linked manner.[11] New imaging techniques such as Positron Emission Tomography (PET) scanning are providing information about the parts of the brain which are involved in the perception of pain.

There will not be a single pathophysiological explanation for non-acute pain. All pains are not the same. Patients with the same apparent cause can present with very different pains. Lack of understanding of all the mechanisms renders selection of therapies more difficult.

PREVENTION

The small trial reported by Bach and colleagues provided a tantalizing suggestion that pre-operative epidural block could prevent the development of post-amputation pains.[12] Jahangiri and colleagues have demonstrated that peri-operative epidural infusion of diamorphine, clonidine and bupivacaine reduces the incidence of phantom pain after amputation.[13] The pre-emptive story is not confined to post-surgical pains. Early rehabilitation prevents the development of chronic disability following an episode of acute back pain.[14] The use of sympathetic blocks within 2 months of an attack of acute herpes zoster has been claimed to reduce the incidence of post-herpetic neuralgia but the evidence is based on retrospective data. Because of the natural history of the disease a very large multi-centre trial is needed to resolve this question.

ASSESSMENT

Many patients with non-acute pain have already been extensively and expensively investigated before referral to a pain specialist and it may be important to stop the fruitless search for a 'cause' of the pain. Over the years various devices have been used to measure or assess pain. There has recently been interest in the use of dynamometric techniques such as isokinetic measurements of spinal movements but the validity of this approach requires rigorous evaluation.[15] Quantitative sensory testing has been developed to test the perception thresholds for different sensory modalities in patients with neurogenic pain. It is difficult to quantify the subjective experience of pain: distress and functional disability can be measured more easily.[16] There is still uncertainty about the validity of many of the methods of assessment and we await further research in this area. Main and colleagues, in 1991, argued for simpler and more focused types of psychological tests when assessing pain and disability.[17]

In some centres, intravenous tests have been employed to aid diagnosis and selection of therapy.[18,19] Lignocaine blocks sodium channels and so could suppress ectopic impulses in damaged nerves. Phentolamine is an alpha-adrenergic receptor blocker so could, in theory, be effective in sympathetically maintained pain. Fentanyl, a mu-opioid receptor agonist, can reveal whether the pain is opioid sensitive when long term opioid therapy is being considered. Diagnostic nerve blocks are sometimes used but caution is advised in interpreting the results because of the high incidence of false positive and false negative responses. The placebo response may account for many false positives. Local anaesthetic blocks may also be poor prognostic indicators of the response to surgical or chemical neuroablation.[20]

CRITICAL APPRAISAL OF THERAPY

A review of recent advances in non-acute pain might be expected to reveal new drugs, new routes of administration, new nerve blocks and new methods of neuroablation. Unfortunately the major advances in the basic sciences have not been reflected by major improvements in the clinical management of non-acute pain and we are still unable to help a significant group of patients.

Today we are amused by 19th century techniques such as metallotherapy, blue light rays, audioanalgesia and mesmerism. What will the next century make of some of the methods in use in the 1990s? New treatments have been introduced into practice before adequate evaluation. Uncontrolled case reports advertise methods which gain a firm foothold in the mythology of pain management long before any controlled trials. To justify continued use of a treatment we must have positive evidence of a positive effect derived from randomized controlled trials (RCT) or from systematic reviews of the literature. Pain clinicians need to accept that validity should be based on scientific rigour rather than on reputation or seniority. There is an urgent need to improve the methods by which surgery and high technology methods are evaluated.[21]

The formulation of everything from individual therapy to broad health policy must be based on the evidence of scientific research. The Cochrane Collaboration has proposed a scheme to prepare and maintain systematic, up-to-date reviews of all the relevant RCTs in particular medical fields.[22] Sackett and his colleagues, in 1991, suggested guidelines for critical appraisal of the medical literature in order to distinguish useful from useless or even harmful therapy and the randomized controlled trial is a key feature.[23] Application of these guidelines to the clinical pain literature would leave us with a very brief review indeed!

APPROPRIATENESS OF CARE

Measuring the appropriateness of various treatments is a major problem in the management of non-acute pain.[24] Management may sometimes be unhelpful or even harmful. Pither and Nicholas examined 89 patients attending a pain management programme and reported that 66% were receiving inappropriate analgesics, 54% were given inappropriate sedatives and tranquillisers, 60% had been over-investigated, 70% had been given inappropriate explanations of their pain, 61% had been encouraged to rest, and 40% had been referred to a psychiatrist.[25]

The relevance of much of the published research in non-acute pain is greatly diminished by the failure to use standard entry and outcome criteria. The International Association for the Study of Pain (IASP) Classification of Chronic Pain provides standard descriptions of chronic pain syndromes and standard definitions of pain terms.[1] Even in the clinical setting the selection of optimal therapy is impeded by the difficulties in assessing outcome.[26]

MEDICATION

Major advances in the basic sciences promised exciting new targetted analgesics but these new weapons have not arisen. The standard analgesics are still variations on willowbark, non steroidal anti-inflammatory drugs (NSAIDs) and poppy (opioids). The method by which these drugs are used may have improved the management of acute pain and cancer pain but not non-acute pain. Of the co-analgesic drugs amitriptyline – an old antidepressant – and carbamazepine – an old anticonvulsant – are still market leaders. A vast range of medication has been used in the treatment of non-acute pain.

The multiplicity of neurochemicals and receptors types involved in nociception suggest many potential targets.[27,28] Opioids act on mu, kappa and delta receptors but kappa and delta agonists are not yet in clinical use. Other potential analgesics include: bradykinin antagonist, substance P antagonist, neurokinin antagonist, cholecystokinin A and B antagonists, calcitonin gene related peptide antagonist, enkephalinase inhibitor, adenosine analogues, galanin agonist, glutamate and aspartate. Ocreotide is a somatostatin analogue which has been suggested as a potent analgesic especially for burning pain and hyperaesthesia.[29] Sumatriptan is a 5-hydroxytryptamine (5HT) 1A receptor agonist which is effective in the treatment of migraine – a 'chronic recurrent acute pain'.

Opioids

Controversy continues over the long term use of opioids in patients with opioid sensitive non-malignant pain.[30,31] The use of opioids should only be considered if other medication has failed and proper trials (e.g. intravenous tests) indicate an unequivocal response to the opioid.[32] Opioids may be appropriate in a patient with spinal cord injury and inappropriate in a patient with atypical facial pain or a history of drug abuse. Side effects and dependence will occur in most patients and tolerance may develop. Psychological dependence is almost never observed in patients with ongoing opioid sensitive pain.[30]

Neuropathic pain and incident pain due to bone secondaries responds poorly or not at all to opioids. Nerve damage may result in a loss of opioid receptors and neurochemicals such as cholecystokinin may interfere with opioid receptors. McQuay and his colleagues described a technique for assessing opioid sensitivity of chronic pain of different aetiologies using patient-controlled analgesia.[33] Nociceptive pain responded better but some patients with neuropathic pain still experienced benefit. Rowbotham and his colleagues demonstrated that some patients with postherpetic neuralgia will obtain relief when given opioids.[34]

In some patients the metabolism of morphine produces an unusually high proportion of morphine 3-glucuronide compared with morphine 6-glucuronide. The 6-glucuronide is a potent analgesic but the 3-glucuronide is inactive or even antagonistic and consequently opioid unresponsiveness may occur. This has been called paradoxical pain. The actual existence of this phenomenon is disputed.[35] However, paradoxic hyperalgesia has been reported in a patient on very high epidural morphine dose.[36] Methadone is not metabolized in the same way as morphine and may be the drug of choice for patients suffering from paradoxical pain.[37]

New sustained-release preparations of morphine and dihydrocodeine have been developed.[38] The morphine preparation contains polymer-coated sustained release pellets. Tramadol is a new mu opioid agonist, with action on monoamine reuptake as well, and results of good trials are awaited. Transdermal fentanyl offers an option for cancer pain. Butorphanol is marketed in the USA in a nasal spray for the relief of migraine.

There is uncertainty about the appropriateness of spinal opioids for chronic non-malignant pain. Abram states that chronic non-malignant pain is more difficult to control with spinal opioids than cancer pain.[39] The suggested indications in cancer pain are tolerance, unreliable absorption by normal routes, unacceptable side effects and the need for drug combinations such as opioid and local anaesthetic to control neuropathic pain or pathological fracture. For a review of the pharmacology see Yaksh.[40] Epidural bupivacaine-opioid infusion is an effective technique for certain cancer patients with refractory pain.[36,41]

Ambulatory infusion devices have allowed cancer patients greater mobility. Other medication such as an antiemetic can be included. The infusion may be subcutaneous, intravenous, spinal, or intraventricular.[42]

There is greater appreciation of the neuropsychiatric toxicity of the opioids and other medication in cancer patients. Psychostimulants such as methylphenidate have been used as adjuvant analgesics. The drugs may potentiate opioid analgesics, counteract opioid induced sedation and cognitive impairment and thus allow dose escalation in difficult pain problems.[43]

Non-steroidal anti-inflammatory drugs

NSAIDs block the action of cyclo-oxygenase upon arachnidonic acid and impede the production of prostanoids (e.g. prostaglandins), which act to sensitize peripheral nociceptors to the excitatory neurochemicals (e.g. bradykinin). In non-acute pain there is rarely a continuing peripheral source of nociceptive stimulation. NSAIDs may be useful in chronic musculo-skeletal pains but are associated with an increased risk of peptic ulcer. Langman and colleagues concluded that ibuprofen and diclofenac carried the lowest risk for gastric bleeding.[44] In a preliminary study Vanos and colleagues report on intravenous regional blocks using ketorolac for reflex sympathetic dystrophy.[45]

Co-analgesics/adjuvants

A wide range of other drugs has been claimed to be effective in non-acute pain but convincing evidence from proper trials is lacking. For a comprehensive review of adjuvants/co-analgesics with critical analysis of the evidence for efficacy see Portenoy.[46]

Tricyclic antidepressants act by enhancement of noradrenergic and serotonergic mechanisms and are effective for neuropathic pain, central pain, atypical facial pain, tension headache, and some musculoskeletal pains.[47] The analgesic effect is separate from the antidepressant effect and occurs with much lower doses. McQuay and his colleagues, in 1993, demonstrated a dose-response for analgesia, and side effects that were unrelated to mood elevation.[48] Amitriptyline, desipramine and maprotiline have been subjected to controlled trials in postherpetic neuralgia and painful diabetic neuropathy. Leijon and Bovie found that amitriptyline was superior to placebo and carbamazepine in central post stroke pain.[49] Dothiepin has been used in atypical facial pain.

Carbamazepine and phenytoin block sodium channels and so depress excitatory transmission. The anticonvulsants are useful for trigeminal neuralgia, diabetic neuropathy and other conditions in which neural damage manifests as epileptiform bursts of spontaneous lightning or shooting pain. Oxcarbazepine has been used for trigeminal neuralgia.[50]

Benzodiazepines such as clonazepam, alprazolam and clobazam are claimed to be helpful in certain neuropathic pains but there is little convincing evidence of major inherent analgesic activity. Intrathecal midazolam may act on gamma amino-butyric acid (GABA) receptors and has been used for cancer pain.[51]

Intravenous lignocaine has been suggested for neuropathic pain but in a randomized controlled trial in neuropathic cancer pain. Bruera and his colleagues were unable to demonstrate any analgesic effect of this technique.[52] Rowbotham's group demonstrated effectiveness of intravenous lignocaine in postherpetic neuralgia.[53] There are also controlled studies in diabetic neuropathy. Uncertainty remains over the value of intravenous local anaesthetics in central pain syndromes. Anti-arrhythmia drugs such as mexiletine and flecainide are used for neuropathic pain.[54-56]

Adrenergic blockers such as phenoxybenzamine, phentolamine and prazosin, as well as corticosteroids and many other drugs have been recommended for sympathetically maintained pain.[57] Guanethidine and bretylium are used in an intravenous regional technique. Adrenergic agonists such as clonidine and medetomidine have been used in a range of different pain conditions.[58,59] Intravenous calcitonin has been used for phantom limb pain. Naloxone has been claimed to be effective in central pain syndromes but this claim is debated. Calcium channel blockers such as nifedipine and diltiazem have been suggested for peripheral neuropathic pain. The bisphosphonate, clodronate, produced a beneficial effect in a randomized trial in patients with painful skeletal metastases resulting from breast cancer.[60] Baclofen, a GABA mimergic agent, is also used for neuropathic lancinating pain and by continuous intrathecal infusion in the management of painful spastic paresis in patients with spinal cord injury or multiple sclerosis.[61] Ketamine is a NMDA (N-methyl-D-aspartate) receptor antagonist which has been used in the treatment of neuropathic pain.[62] Stannard and Porter reported successful use of ketamine in three patients suffering from phantom limb pain.[63] Notcutt describes a new use of ketamine (given in a dose of 1.5 mg/kg) in easing the pain during transport of patients with painful spinal metastases.[64]

Capsaicin selectively depletes substance P from terminal afferents. Watson has reviewed the use of topical capsaicin in a variety of conditions and he concludes that it is generally not satisfactory as a sole therapy although in some cases it may serve as an adjuvant analgesic.[65] The burning sensation produced by the capsaicin has frustrated efforts to conduct double-blind trials.

NEURAL BLOCKADE IN MANAGEMENT OF NON-ACUTE PAIN

The rationale for attacks on the peripheral 'wiring' ignores the likely complex multidimensional pathophysiology of non-acute pain. The substances injected include local anaesthetics, corticosteroids, glycerine, and neurolytic solutions such as phenol or alcohol. Physical methods use cryolesions or radiofrequency thermocoagulation. Sclerosant solutions are claimed to destroy nerves and stimulate the formation of scar tissue. Glycerol suppresses experimental neuroma activity, as does topical corticosteroid.[66] Intracutaneous or subcutaneous injections of sterile water have been claimed to give good results for whiplash and musculoskeletal trigger point pain syndromes but convincing evidence is lacking.

An ultra long-acting local anaesthetic would be useful. Tetrodotoxin is excellent in vitro but toxic in vivo. Current research efforts are aimed at modifying existing drugs to yield new release mechanisms. Release may be delayed by storing the local anaesthetic in a lipid solution. Sustained or prolonged release may come from pellets containing local anaesthetic and biodegradable polymers, lipid encapsulated local anaesthetic or microencapsulated local anaesthetic in crystalline form. Korsten and colleagues reported on the use of a series of injections of *n*-butyl-*p*-aminobenzoate (a congener of benzocaine) in 12 patients with intractable cancer pain.[67] Once established, the sensory block lasted until death in 10 patients for up to 133 days and was not associated with motor block. The mode of action is not clear but further investigation would seem warranted. In a randomized controlled trial in patients with cancer pain, King and colleagues demonstrated prolongation of the anaesthetic effect of epidural bupivacaine up to a mean value of about 12 hours when mixed with 50% glycerine. When given alone 50% glycerine did not produce any analgesic effect.[68]

There are hundreds of published reports on the use of epidural injections for low back pain but few randomized controlled trials. Consequently, we do not possess conclusive scientific evidence about the efficacy or the indications. The prevailing impression suggests that epidural corticosteroids are beneficial for painful radiculopathy where there may be both a mechanical and an inflammatory component.[69] The factors said to be associated with failure of lumbar corticosteroids include: being unemployed because of pain; a duration of symptoms over 6 months; primary diagnosis that is not radiculopathy and smoking.

There is debate over the safety of epidural corticosteroids. The data sheet for depot methylprednisolone states in bold type in two places that the preparation must not be given by the intrathecal route and there is little dispute about this. The data sheet also states that the preparation is not recommended for the epidural route. The controversy was precipitated by Nelson who claimed that the polyethylene glycol in the carrier vehicle could penetrate to the subarachnoid space via the arachnoid villi.[70] In support he quoted a single case report which described localized dural fibrosis in a patient with lumbar disc disease who had received epidural steroids. Cause and effect are not established by this case and there is little supporting evidence. Cicala did not detect any significant difference to controls in the tissue reaction when a single dose of depot methylprednisolone was injected into the epidural space of a rabbit.[71] It is acknowledged that intrathecal depot methylprednisolone injection is potentially harmful and Nelson[70] claims that epidural injection is also dangerous because of the risk of inadvertent dural puncture and subsequent subarachnoid injection of the steroid. Abram and colleagues failed to show any histologic evidence of neurotoxicity following four repeated injections of intrathecal triamcinolone at 5-day intervals in rats.[72]

Facet joint injections and facet joint denervation continue in the repertoire of many pain practitioners.[73] Local anaesthetic blocks of the medial branch of the dorsal rami are claimed to be specific for the diagnosis of cervical zygapophyseal joint pain.[74] Other authors have failed to demonstrate any convincing link between diagnostic lumbar facet joint blocks and the outcome of either surgical fusion or non-operative treatment.[75]

Chemical sympathectomy is an effective treatment for rest pain and skin ulceration due to occlusive vascular disease but of much less benefit for claudication. It is difficult to predict outcome prior to the block. Altomare and colleagues have described the use of an acetylcholine sweatspot test before and after sympathectomy.[76] Patients with hyperhidrosis may be referred for sympathetic nerve blocks. Before neuroablative sympathetic blocks are considered the patient should have a thorough trial of conservative treatment. Endoscopic transthoracic sympathectomy of the upper limb is a safe and effective alternative to open cervical sympathectomy in the management of hyperhidrosis as well as vasospastic conditions and sympathetically maintained pain.[77] Stellate ganglion block was used for intractable angina in the days before coronary artery bypass surgery. Endoscopic transthoracic sympathectomy has recently been described as being of benefit after an uncontrolled trial in a group of 24 patients with severe angina.[78]

Neurolytic coeliac plexus block is widely used for pain due to pancreatic cancer but Sharfman and Walsh have called for a rigorous evaluation of the technique.[79] Mercadante compared coeliac plexus block with conventional analgesics in a series of 20 patients and showed beneficial effects of both approaches, although there was a higher incidence of side effects with the analgesic group.[80] Pain from chronic pancreatitis does not respond as well to coeliac plexus block. The use of computerised tomography (CT) scanning has been claimed to improve the safety and effectiveness of the block.[81] Kirvela and colleagues describe the advantages of using ultrasonic guidance for lumbar sympathetic and coeliac plexus block.[82] Davies reviewed 2730 neurolytic coeliac plexus blocks and concluded that major complications (paraplegia with or without loss of sphincter function) happened once per 683 blocks.[83]

Bilateral chemical sympathectomy has been claimed to be an effective treatment for rectal tenesmoid pain due to pelvic carcinoma.[84] Superior hypogastric plexus block for pelvic cancer pain targets the sympathetic plexus which lies anterior to the sacral promontory.[85] Block of the ganglion impar has been used for perineal pain in cancer. Zorn and colleagues describe a periprostatic block of the pelvic plexus using a needle guided by transrectal ultrasound in patients with chronic orchidalgia.[86] Chronic testicular pain often fails to respond to a wide range of therapies and even orchidectomy may not to provide relief.

Intravenous regional sympathetic blocks (Bier's block) have enjoyed great popularity for many years. The effects of bretylium and guanethidine on peripheral sympathetic mechanisms were recorded as long ago as 1963.[87] There is a lack of evidence from methodologically sound randomized controlled trials to support the contention that intravenous guanethidine is of great value in so-called reflex sympathetic dystrophy.[88]

Post thoracotomy cancer pain has been managed with interpleural bupivacaine for over 7 weeks.[89] Interpleural blocks have also been used for cancer and chronic pancreatitis. Pleural injection of phenol has been suggested for pain associated with oesophageal cancer. Kirvela and Antila carried out a retrospective review of 281 thoracic paravertebral blocks performed for chronic postoperative pain and suggest that it is a reliable and safe technique for unilateral pain.[90]

STIMULATION-PRODUCED ANALGESIA

The clinical response to acupuncture and TENS (transcutaneous electrical nerve stimulation) is variable and unpredictable but some patients do gain significant benefit without serious adverse effects.[91] Headaches, musculoskeletal disorders, and some neuropathic pains may respond well to these techniques. Transcutaneous electrical spinal stimulation is a new technique which awaits proper evaluation. Deluze and colleagues reported a three weeks' double-blind randomized trial of electroacupuncture in fibromyalgia.[92] The results showed a significant improvement in the active treatment group. In a randomized controlled trial Vincent compared true and sham acupuncture in migraine and showed benefits for true acupuncture.[93]

Chronic pain resulting from incomplete deafferentation may respond to neurostimulation. Pain following peripheral nerve injury may respond to peripheral nerve stimulation in about 51% of cases.[94] Other cases of nerve injury may respond to peripheral nerve repair.[95] It is now obvious that pain following peripheral nerve injury does not respond regularly or reliably to sympathetic blockade.

Spinal cord stimulation (SCS) has been claimed to help arachnoiditis, postlaminectomy syndrome, peripheral vascular disease, peripheral nerve injury, post amputation pain, painful peripheral neuropathy, spinal cord injury, and intractable angina. The exact mode of action of spinal cord stimulation remains a mystery. The benefit in peripheral vascular disease and intractable angina may relate to physiological changes quite separate from pain mechanisms.[96] Gybels concludes that SCS is not a simple intervention but a time consuming and rather expensive technique.[94] Deep-brain stimulation is generally applied through an electrode implanted in the periventricular grey matter of the posterior end of the third ventricle or in the sensory thalamus, but why electrical stimulation of the brain suppresses chronic pain is not well understood.

NEUROSURGERY

Neurosurgical techniques are now used less often following the realization that cutting the nervous system anywhere is rarely the answer to non-acute pain.[97,98] Modern techniques such as dorsal-root entry-zone lesioning are indicated in conditions such as brachial plexus avulsion. Stuart and Crammond reported on 273 patients who underwent percutaneous cervical cordotomy for pain of malignant origin.[99] They concluded that this remains a valuable technique particularly for patients with lung cancer and mesothelioma. Gybels agrees that the operation is useful for unilateral pain in the extremities and trunk but he observes that percutaneous anterolateral cordotomy is not an easy procedure and requires continuing practice in order to maintain consistently good results.[94] Selective posterior rhizotomy may be considered for Pancoast's syndrome. Spinal surgery should always be considered in the treatment of metastatic back pain,[100] and pain resulting from long bone metastases should be managed with operative immobilization where instability exists.[101]

PHYSICAL THERAPY

In a randomized trial[102] for patients with persistent back and neck pain Koes and colleagues reported that manipulative therapy and physiotherapy were superior to general practitioner or placebo treatment at one-year follow up, but another study found manipulation only useful for acute episodes of back pain and of very little benefit in chronic back pain.[103]

In the UK the Clinical Standard Advisory Group Committee on Back Pain[104] has published an epidemiology review and management guidelines which address the spreading epidemic of low back pain. The management guidelines highlight the need for active rehabilitation within the first six weeks of onset in order to prevent long term pain and disability. Frost and colleagues have conducted a randomized controlled trial[105] to evaluate a fitness programme for patients with chronic low back pain and they showed that moderately disabled patients with chronic low back pain who attend a back school and fitness programme benefit more in the short and long term than patients who attend a back school and exercise independently at home. Significant differences existed between the groups in measures of disability, self efficacy and walking distance as well as in the sensory and affective components of pain. This trial demonstrates the need to assess a wide range of measures and not just pain alone.[106] In another study, 87% of 116 patients who participated in a functional restoration programme were working at 2-year follow up compared with only 41% of the 72 patients in the untreated control group.[14] Rehabilitation programmes can be vital even for cases with irreversible damage such as avulsion lesions of the brachial plexus.[107]

PSYCHOLOGY

The psychological dimensions of non-acute pain become more important with increasing chronicity whether or not organic disease is present.[108] Patients with the same degree of tissue damage respond differently and this is often due to psychological factors. The presence of a significant psychological component is suggested by: pain persisting beyond expected healing time; disparity between objective findings and functional disability; signs and symptoms of psychiatric abnormality; excessive dependence on health care facilities; excessive dependence on medication.

Many patients with non-acute pain have been in the traditional medical system for a long time. The expectation of doctor and patient is that the history, examination and investigation will lead to a diagnosis which will lead to a specific treatment and cure. The traditional disease model works for acute pain but not for non-acute pain hence relief is not forthcoming. The patient experiences increasing helplessness, hopelessness and dependence, depression, social withdrawal, and family breakdown. As pain persists, the more it and associated behaviours are susceptible to the effects of learning and experience.[109] The behaviours may be reinforced by powerful influences in the environment. For example inactivity is reinforced by avoidance of work. Inactivity leads to weakness, lack of fitness and more pain. Fear and misunderstanding of pain leads to decreased activity and an increase in unhelpful and negative beliefs – which in turn reinforce pain behaviour. For example the belief (cognition) that 'I will damage myself if I climb stairs.' evokes the response (behaviour) of rest and avoidance of activity. Excess disability becomes the major problem of many patients with non-acute pain.

It is important to recognize that not all pain behaviour is inappropriate or 'pathological'. The patients who will benefit from psychological approaches are those in whom the behaviours are exaggerated or clearly inappropriate. Cognitive behavioural approaches aim to achieve the best possible level of physical and emotional function within the confines of the condition. Pain reduction is not an aim but may follow the improvement in function. Therapy involves behaviour modification, physical rehabilitation, medication reduction, education, cognitive therapy, group discussion, relaxation techniques, family therapy and individual psychological support. It is important to decrease catastrophizing and to increase perceived patient control over pain. Participation of the spouse or family is vital.

Outcome studies which analyse pain, function, psychology and economics suggest that these programmes are effective.[110] Williams and colleagues demonstrated increased activity, decreased medication and decreased reported pain experience.[111] Patients are more likely to return to work and to normal day-to-day activity. Quality of life improves. Peters and colleagues have demonstrated the significant cost benefits of a pain management programme in returning patients to useful employment.[112] There is a need to improve pre-treatment assessment in order to match patients to the appropriate treatment package. There are other questions. What is the optimal time point for intervention? What parts of the programme are important? How do we manage patients resistant to treatment? How do we ensure adherence to the programme? As the programme increases in complexity then compliance falls off dramatically!

SOME SPECIFIC MANAGEMENT PROBLEMS

Chronic and recurrent pain in childhood is now receiving considerable attention. Common conditions include recurrent abdominal pain, headaches and musculoskeletal pains. Psychological factors may play an important part.[113]

Post amputation pain syndromes including phantom pain and stump pain are very common but there is no reliable treatment.[114] This is a classic example of a chronic pain syndrome where attacks on the periphery are often fruitless serving as evidence that the pathophysiological disturbance has migrated centrally although the initial injury was clearly peripheral.

Chronic pelvic pain is a very common complaint in gynaecological practice. It has been suggested that up to 12% of hysterectomies are performed for pelvic pain and that the pain often continues unabated. The treatment of chronic pelvic pain without obvious pathology remains unsatisfactory but psychological techniques have benefited some.[115]

Chronic perineal pain remains a difficult management problem.[116] Sacral cysts were linked to perineal pain in one report.[117] Delayed onset of perineal pain after rectal resection is usually associated with tumour recurrence.[118]

Back pain. Recent reviews have highlighted the complexity of chronic low back pain.[119,120] The new IASP classification[1] emphasizes the important distinction between spinal pain (with or without referred pain) and radicular pain. The term sciatica is an anachronism and should not be used.

Osteoporosis is probably the most common skeletal disorder in the world and is a frequent cause of pain and disability, especially in older women. The bisphosphonates may aid in the prevention and treatment of osteoporosis although the effect on fracture rate is uncertain.[121] The management of the incident pain which results from fractures of an osteoporotic spine is still a major problem and is often unsatisfactory in older patients who may be intolerant of powerful medication and corsets whilst being incapable of regaining muscle strength.

Whiplash is a term which has been replaced by acceleration deceleration injury of the neck or cervical spine injury.[122] Pain will persist for over six months in about 25% and it is likely that by this time psychological, behavioural and economic factors may complicate the original injury. No single therapy can be recommended.

Spinal cord injury. There are 20 000 patients in the UK with spinal cord injury and it has been estimated that 50% suffer from persistent pain which in many cases is difficult to manage. Pain is more common after incomplete injuries to the cord and is typically neuropathic but the pain may also be due to associated musculoskeletal problems such as vertebral instability. In general a multidisciplinary rehabilitation orientated approach, including psychological techniques, is most likely to benefit these patients.[123]

Reflex sympathetic dystrophy (RSD) was regarded as a very unsatisfactory term since many of the cases to which it was applied either did not exhibit any signs of sympathetic disturbance and dystrophy or, even if they did, they failed to respond to sympathetic block. A new term, Complex Regional Pain Syndrome (CRPS) Type I (Table 9.1) should replace RSD.[1] Causalgia is CRPS Type II (Table 9.2). Sympathetically maintained pain may be found in association with either of these syndromes. Irrespective of the name, management remains difficult in many cases. Physical therapy may be the most important treatment. Other therapies include somatic nerve blocks, plexus or epidural infusions, sympathetic nerve blocks, intravenous regional blocks, surgical sympathectomy, TENS and spinal cord stimulation, and a vast array of medication: corticosteroids, tricyclics, prazocin, phenoxybenzamine, nifedipine, labetalol, propranolol, clonidine and topical capsaicin.[57]

Sickle cell disease – These patients frequently have non-acute pain as well as the recurrent episodes of acute pain during a crisis; up to 20% have three to 10 severe episodes per year; 50% have one severe crisis per year.[124]

Human immunodeficiency virus disease is presenting new problems of non-acute pain.[125]

A number of what might be loosely described as 'fashionable conditions' present in the pain clinic. Patients with the chronic fatigue syndrome may complain of widespread muscle pain. Management is difficult and a substantial proportion of patients may remain functionally impaired.[126] The very existence of repetitive strain injury is challenged.[127] A number of authors dispute the existence of fibromyalgia as a distinct disease entity and suggest that the tender points, which are a crucial part of the diagnosis of fibromyalgia, are a measure of general distress and although related to pain they are associated separately with fatigue and depression.[128,129]

COMPENSATION AND DISABILITY

It is important to distinguish between disability and impairment. As many as one-third of chronic pain patients will have no objective findings of somatic disease.[130] There is evidence that compensation issues may interfere with

Table 9.1 Complex Regional Pain Syndrome – Type I[1]

Diagnostic criteria

1. Initiating noxious event or cause of immobilization
2. Continuing pain, allodynia, or hyperalgesia – pain is disproportionate to inciting event
3. At some time – oedema, changes in skin blood flow, abnormal sudomotor activity
4. No other condition to account for the degree of pain and dysfunction

Criteria 2–4 must be satisfied.

Table 9.2 Complex Regional Pain Syndrome – Type II[1]

Diagnostic criteria

1. Continuing pain, allodynia, or hyperalgesia after a nerve injury
2. At some time – oedema, changes in skin blood flow, abnormal sudomotor activity
3. No other condition to account for the degree of pain and dysfunction

All three criteria must be satisfied.

evaluation and treatment of chronic pain patients.[131] Pain clinicians are often asked to prepare medical reports on patients with persisting pain and disability some time after an injury or illness and when the issue of pending compensation acts as a cloud to rational resolution. These patients may remain disabled after the litigation is finished.

CONCLUSION

Today's major challenge is changing doctors' perception of pain and methods of treatment, not just amongst pain clinicians but in the wider medical community.[132] John J Bonica and Sampson Lipton both died during 1994 after lifetimes devoted to helping patients with non-acute pain. The major recent advances in non-acute pain management during their lives were the increased awareness of the size of the problem and the recognition of the need to provide specific services to manage these patients. Management must take account of the multidimensional nature of non-acute pain. The biopsychosocial model is of more relevance than the traditional medical model. The future may bring more specific treatments based on an improved understanding of the specific pathophysiology of different pain syndromes but for the moment there are no 'magic bullets'. Optimal use of current drugs and techniques will produce satisfactory relief for many patients.

KEY POINTS FOR CLINICAL PRACTICE

- The pathophysiology of non-acute pain is likely to be multidimensional in many cases.
- No two pains are the same and individualization of management is essential.
- A combination of treatments (multimodal therapy) is necessary in most cases.
- Use simultaneous rather than sequential application of multimodal therapy.
- Patient participation in decision making and management is essential.
- Use the biopsychosocial model rather than a traditional disease model.
- Pay attention to disability as well as the symptom of pain.
- Whenever possible choose therapy which has been subjected to critical appraisal.

REFERENCES

1. Merskey H. Bogduk N. Classification of chronic pain: descriptions of chronic pain syndromes and definitions of pain terms. 2nd edn. IASP Press, Seattle, 1994
2. Bowsher D, Rigge M, Sopp L. Prevalence of chronic pain in a British population – a telephone survey of 1037 households. The Pain Clinic 1991; 4: 223–230

3. McQuay H J, Machin L, Moore R A. Chronic non-malignant pain: a population prevalence study. Practitioner 1985; 229: 1109–1111
4. Bonica J J. Past and current status of pain research and therapy. Sem Anesth 1986; 5; 82–89
5. Clinical Standard Advisory Group. Epidemiology Review: The Epidemiology and Cost of Back Pain. Her Majesty's Stationery Office, London, 1994
6. James F R, Large R G. Chronic pain and the use of health services. New Zealand Med J 1992; 105: 196–198
7. Davies H T O, Crombie I K , Macrae W A. Waiting in pain. Delays between referral and consulation in outpatient pain clinics. Anaesthesia 1994; 49: 661–665
8. Melzack R, Wall P D. Pain mechanisms: a new theory. Science 1965; 150: 971–979
9. McQuay H J, Dickenson A H. Implications of nervous system plasticity for pain management. Anaesthesia 1990; 45: 101–102
10. Fields H L. Is there a facilitating component to central pain modulation. APS J 1992; 1: 139–141
11. Flor H, Birbaumer N. Acquisition of chronic pain: psychophysiological mechanisms, APS J 1994; 3: 119–127
12. Bach S, Noreng M F, Tjellden N U. Phantom limb pain in amputees during the first 12 months following limb amputation after pre-operative lumbar epidural blockade. Pain 1988; 33: 297–301
13. Jahangiri M, Bradley J W P, Jayatunga A P, Dark C H. Prevention of phantom pain after major lower limb amputation by epidural infusion of diamorphine, clonidine and bupivacaine. Ann R Coll Surg Engl 1994; 76: 324–326
14. Mayer T G, Gatchel R J, Mayer H, Kishino N D, Keeley J, Mooney V. A prospective two year study of functional restoration in industrial low back injury; an objective assessment procedure. JAMA 1987; 258: 1763–1767
15. Jayson M I V. Trauma, back pain, malingering, and compensation. BMJ 1993; 305: 7–8
16. Waddell G, Pilowsky I, Bond M R. Clinical assessment and interpretation of abnormal illness behaviour in low back pain. Pain 1989; 39: 41–53
17. Main C J, Evans P J D, Whitehead R C. An investigation of personality structure and other psychological features in patients presenting with low-back pain: a critique of the MMPI. In: Bond M R, Charlton J E, Woolf C J (eds) Proceedings of the VIth World Congress on Pain. Elsevier, Amsterdam,1991: pp 207–217
18. Raja S, Treede R, Davis K, Campbell J. Systemic alpha-adrenergic blockade with phentolamine: a diagnostic test for sympathetically maintained pain. Anesthesiology 1991; 74: 691–698
19. Arner S. Intravenous phentolamine test: diagnostic and prognostic use in reflex sympathetic dystrophy. Pain 1991; 46: 17–22
20. Boas R A. Nerve blocks in the diagnosis of low back pain. Neurosurg Clin 1991; 2: 807–816
21. Large R, Peters J. A critical appraisal of outcome of multidisciplinary pain clinic treatments. In: Bond M R, Charlton J E, Woolf C J (eds) Proceedings of the VIth World Congress on Pain. Amsterdam, Elsevier, 199: pp 417–427
22. Chalmers I, Haynes B. Reporting, updating, and correcting systematic reviews of the effects of health care. B M J 1994; 309: 862–865
23. Sackett D L, Haynes R B, Guyatt G H, Tugewell P. Clinical Epidemiology: A Basic Science for Clinical Medicine. 2nd edn. Little Brown, Boston, 1991: p 193
24. Hicks N R. Some observations on attempts to measure appropriateness of care. BMJ 1994; 309: 730–733
25. Pither C E, Nicholas M K. The identification of iatrogenic factors in the development of chronic pain syndromes: abnormal treatment behaviour? In: Bond M R, Charlton J E, Woolf C J (eds) Proceedings of the VIth World Congress on Pain. Elsevier, Amsterdam, 1991: pp 429–434
26. Turk D C, Rudy T E, Sorkin B A. Neglected topics in chronic pain treatment outcome studies: determination of success. Pain 1993; 53: 3–16
27. Basbaum A I, Besson J-M. (eds) Towards a New Pharmacotherapy of Pain. Wiley, Chichester, 1991

28. Besson J-M. The pharmacology of pain: twenty five years of hope, despair and hope. In: Gebhart G F, Hammond D L, Jensen T S (eds) Proceedings of the 7th World Congress on Pain. IASP Press, Seattle, 1994: pp 23–39
29. Mercadante S. The role of octreotide in palliative care. J Pain Sympt Man 1994; 9: 406–411
30. Portenoy R K, Foley K M. Chronic use of opioid analgesics in non-malignant pain: report of 38 cases. Pain 1986; 25: 171–186
31. Wall P D. Neuropathic pain. Pain 1990; 43: 267–268
32. Jadad A R, Carroll D, Glynn C J et al. Morphine responsiveness in chronic pain: double blind randomised cross over study with PCA. Lancet 1992; 33: 1367–1371
33. McQuay H J, Jadad A R, Carroll D et al. Opioid sensitivity of chronic pain: a patient-controlled analgesia method. Anaesthesia 1992; 47: 757–767
34. Rowbotham M C, Reisner-Keller L A, Fields H L. Both intravenous lidocaine and morphine reduce the pain of postherpetic neuralgia. Neurology 1991; 41: 1024–1028
35. Bowsher D. Paradoxical pain. BMJ 1993 306: 473
36. Hogan Q, Haddox J D, Abram S, Weissman D, Taylor M L, Janjan N. Epidural opiates and local anesthetics for the management of cancer pain. Pain 1991; 46: 271–279
37. Davis C L, Hardy J R. Palliative care. BMJ 1994; 308: 1359–1362
38. Gourlay G K, Plummer J L, Cherry D A, Onley M M. A comparison of Kapanol (a new sustained release morphine formulation), MST Continus, and morphine solution in cancer patients: pharmacokinetic aspects of morphine and morphine metabolites. In: Gebhart G F, Hammond D L, Jensen T S (eds) Proceedings of the 7th World Congress on Pain. IASP Press, Seattle, 1994: pp 631–643
39. Abram S E. Advances in chronic pain management since gate control. Regional Anesthesia 1993: 18: 66–81
40. Yaksh T L. The spinal pharmacology of acutely and chronically administered opioids. J Pain Sympt Man 1992; 7: 356–361
41. Du Pen S, Kharasch E D, Williams A, et al. Chronic epidural bupivacaine-opioid infusion in intractable cancer pain. Pain 1992; 49: 293–300
42. Bruera E. Ambulatory infusion devices in the continuing care of patients with advanced disease. J Pain Sympt Man. 1990; 5: 287–296
43. Bruera E, Watanabe S. Psychostimulants as adjuvant analgesics. J Pain Sympt Man 1994; 9: 412–415
44. Langman M J S, Weil J, Wainwright P et al. Risks of peptic ulcer associated with individual non-steroidal anti-inflammatory drugs. Lancet 1994; 343: 1075–1078
45. Vanos D N, Ramamurthy S, Hoffman J. Intravenous regional block using ketorolac: preliminary results in the treatment of reflex sympathetic dystrophy. Anesth Analg 1992; 74: 139–141
46. Portenoy R K. Adjuvant analgesics in pain management. In: Doyle D, Hanks G W C, MacDonald N (eds) Oxford Textbook of Palliative Medicine. University Press, Oxford, 1993; pp 187–203
47. Watson C P N. Antidepressant drugs as adjuvant analgesics. J Pain Sympt Man 1994; 9: 392–405
48. McQuay H J, Carroll D, Glynn C J. Dose-response for analgesic effect of amitriptyline in chronic pain. Anaesthesia 1993; 48: 281–285
49. Leijon G, Boivie J. Central post-stroke pain – a controlled trial of amitriptyline and carbamazepine. Pain 1989; 36: 27–36
50. Zakrzewska J M, Patsalos P N. Oxcarbazepine: a new drug in the management of intractable trigeminal neuralgia. J Neurol, Neurosurg Psych 1989; 52: 472–476
51. Edwards M, Serrao J M, Gent J P et al. On the mechanism by which midazolam causes spinally mediated analgesia. Anesthesiology 1990; 73: 273–277
52. Bruera E, Ripamonti C, Brenneis C et al. A randomised double-blind crossover trial of intravenous lidocaine in the treatment of neuropathic cancer pain. J Pain Sympt Man 1992; 7: 138–140
53. Rowbotham M C, Reisner-Keller L A, Fields H L. Both intravenous lidocaine and morphine reduce the pain of postherpetic neuralgia. Neurology 1991; 41: 1024–1028

54. Hanks G W. Opioid responsive and opioid non-responsive pain in cancer. Br Med Bull 1991; 47: 718–731
55. Dejgard A, Petersen P, Kastrup J. Mexiletine for treatment of chronic painful diabetic neuropathy. Lancet 1988; 1: 9–11
56. Glazer S, Portenoy R K. Systemic local anesthetics in pain control. J Pain Sympt Man 1991; 6: 30–39
57. Charlton J E. Reflex sympathetic dystrophy. non-invasive methods of treatment. In: Stanton-Hicks M, Janig W, Boas R A (eds) Reflex sympathetic dystrophy. Kluwer, Boston, 1990: pp 151–164
58. Nagasaka H, Yaksh T L. Pharmacology of intrathecal adrenergic agonists. Anesthesiology 1990; 73: 1198–1207
59. Kauppilia T, Kemppainene P, Tanila H et al. Effect of systemic medetomidine, an alpha 2 adrenoreceptor agonist, on experimental pain in man. Anesthesiology 1991; 74: 3–8
60. Patterson A H G, Powles T J, Kanis J A et al. Double blind controlled trial of oral clodronate in patients with bone metastaes from breast cancer. J Clin Oncol 1993; 11: 59–65
61. Penn R D, Savoy S M, Corcos D et al. Intrathecal baclofen for severe spinal spasticity. N Engl J Med 1989; 320: 1517–1521
62. Dickenson A H. NMDA receptor antagonists as analgesics. In: Fields H L, Liebeskind J C (eds) Progress in Pain Research and Management. Vol 1. IASP Press, Seattle, 1994: pp 173–187
63. Stannard C F, Porter G E. Ketamine hydrochloride in the treatment of phantom limb pain. Pain 1993; 54: 227–230
64. Notcutt W G. Transporting patients with overwhelming pain. Anaesthesia 1994; 49: 145–147
65. Watson C P N. Topical capsaicin as an adjuvant analgesic. J Pain Sympt Man 1994; 9: 425–433
66. Devor M, Govrin-Lippmann R, Raber P. Corticosteroids suppress ectopic neuronal discharge originating in experimental neuromas. Pain 1985; 22: 127–137
67. Korsten H H M, Ackerman E W, Grouls R J et al. Long-lasting epidural sensory blockade by n-butyl-p-aminobenzoate in the terminally ill intractable cancer pain patient. Anesthesiology 1991; 75: 950–960
68. King H-K, Xiao C-S, Wooten D J. Prolongation of epidural bupivacaine analgesia with glycerin. Canad Anesth Soc J 1993; 40: 431–434
69. Rowlingson J C. Epidural steroids. Do they have a place in management? APS J 1994; 3: 20–27
70. Nelson D A. Dangers from methylprednisolone acetate therapy by intraspinal injection. Arch Neurol 1988; 45: 804–806
71. Cicala R S, Turner R, Moran E et al. Methylprednisolone acetate does not cause inflammatory changes in the epidural space. Anesthesiology 1990; 72: 556–558
72. Abram S E, Marsala M, Yaksh T L. Analgesic and neurotoxic effects of intrathecal steroids in rats. Anesthesiology 1992; 77: A810
73. Stolker R J, Vervest A C M, Groen G J. The management of spinal pain by blockades: a review. Pain 1994; 58: 1–20
74. Barnsley L, Bogduk N. Medial branch blocks are specific for the diagnosis of cervical zygapophyseal joint pain. Regional Anesthesia 1993; 18: 343–350
75. Esses S I, Moro J K. The value of facet joint blocks in patient selection for lumbar fusion. Spine 1993; 18: 185–190
76. Altomare D F, Regina G, Lovreglio R, Memeo V. Acetylcholine sweat test: an effective way to select patients for lumbar sympathectomy. Lancet 1994; 344: 976–978
77. Byrne J, Walsh T N, Hederman W P. Endoscopic transthoracic electrocautery of the sympathetic chain for palmer and axillary hyperhidrosis. Br J Surg 1990; 77: 1040–1049
78. Wettervik C, Claes G, Drott C et al. Endoscopic transthoracic sympathectomy for severe angina. Lancet 1995; 345: 97–98
79. Sharfman W H, Walsh T D. Has the analgesic efficacy of neurolytic celiac plexus block been demonstrated in pancreatic cancer pain? Pain 1990; 41: 267–271

80. Mercadante S. Celiac plexus block versus analgesics in pancreatic cancer pain. Pain 1993; 52: 182–192
81. Brown D L, Moore D C. The use of neurolytic celiac plexus block for pancreatic cancer: anatomy and technique. J Pain Sympt Man 1988; 3: 206–209
82. Kirvela O, Svedstrom E, Lundblom N. Ultrasonic guidance of lumbar sympathetic and coeliac plexus block. A new technique. Regional Anesthesia 1992; 17: 43–46
83. Davies D D. Incidence of major complications of neurolytic coeliac plexus block. J R Soc Med 1993; 86: 264–266
84. Bristow A, Foster J M G. Lumbar sympathectomy in the management of rectal tenesmoid pain. Ann R Coll Surg Engl 1988; 70: 38–39
85. Plancarte R, Amescua C, Patt R B, Aldrete J A. Superior hypogastric plexus block for pelvic cancer pain. Anesthesiology 1990; 73: 236–239
86. Zorn B H, Watson L R, Steers W D. Nerves from pelvic plexus contribute to chronic orchidalgia. Lancet 1994; 343: 1161
87. Cooper C J, Fewings J D, Hodge R L, Whelan R F. Effects of bretylium and guanethidine on human hand and forearm vessels and on their sensitivity to noradrenaline. Br J Pharmacol 1963; 21: 165–173
88. Blanchard J, Ramamurthy S, Walsh N et al. Intravenous regional sympatholysis: a double blind comparison of guanethidine, reserpine, and normal saline. J Pain Sympt Man 1990; 5: 357–361
89. Fineman S P. Long-term post-thoracotomy cancer pain management with interpleural bupivacaine. Anesth Analg 1989; 68: 694–697
90. Kirvela O, Antila H. Thoracic paravertebral block in chronic postoperative pain. Regional Anesthesia 1992; 17: 348–350
91. Johnson M I, Ashton C H, Thompson J W. An in depth study of long term users of transcutaneous electrical nerve stimulation (TENS). Implications for clinical use of TENS. Pain 1991; 44: 221–229
92. Deluze C, Bosia L, Zirbs A et al. Electroacupuncture in fibromyalgia: results of a controlled trial. BMJ 1992; 305: 1249–1252
93. Vincent C A. A controlled trial of the treament of migraine by acupuncture. Clin J Pain 1989; 5: 305–312
94. Gybels J M.Indications for the use of neurosurgical techniques in pain control. In: Bond M R, Charlton J E, Woolf C J (eds) Proceedings of the VIth World Congress on Pain. Elsevier, Amsterdam, 1991: pp 475–482
95. Campbell J N, Raja S N, Meyer R A. Painful sequelae of nerve injury. In: Dubner R, Gebhart G F, Bond M R (eds) Pain Research and Clinical Management, Vol 3. Elsevier, Amsterdam, 1988: pp 135–143
96. Tallis R, Jacobs M, Miles J B. Spinal cord stimulation in peripheral vascular disease. Br J Neurosurg 1992; 6: 101–105
97. Tasker R R. Management of nociceptive, deafferentation and central pain by surgical intervention. In: Fields H L (ed) Pain syndromes in neurology. Butterworths, London, 1990: pp 143–200
98. Loeser J D. Ablative neurosurgical operations. In: Bonica J J (ed) The Management of Pain. 2nd edn. Lea and Febiger, Philadelphia, 1990: pp 2040–2043
99. Stuart G, Crammond T. Role of percutaneous cervical cordotomy for pain of malignant origin. Medical J Australia 1993; 158: 667–670
100. Fallon M T, O'Neill W M. Spinal surgery in the treatment of metastatic back pain. Palliative Medicine 1993; 7: 235–238
101. Chan D, Carter S R, Grimer R J, Sneath R S. Endoprosthetic replacement for bone metastases. Ann R Coll Surg Engl 1992; 74: 13–18
102. Koes B W, Bouter L M, van Mameren H et al. Randomised clinical trial of manipulative therapy and physiotherapy for persistent back and neck complaints: results of one year follow up. BMJ 1992; 304: 601–605
103. Meade T W, Dyer S, Browne W et al. Low back pain of mechanical origin: randomised comparison of chiropractic and hospital outpatient treatment. BMJ 1990; 300: 1431–1437
104. Clinical Standard Advisory Group. Back Pain. Her Majesty's Stationery Office, London, 1994

105. Frost H, Klaber Moffett J A, Moser J S, Fairbank J C T. Randomised controlled trial for evaluation of fitness programme for patients with chronic low back pain. BMJ 1994; 310: 151–154
106. Waddell G. Clinical assessment of lumbar impairment. Clin Orthop Res 1987; 221: 110–120
107. Wynn Parry C B. Pain in avulsion lesions of the brachial plexus Pain 1980; 9: 41–53
108. Sternbach R A. (ed) The Psychology of Pain. 2nd ed. Raven, New York, 1986
109. Fordyce W E. Learning processes in pain. In: The Psychology of Pain. Sternbach R A (ed) Raven, New York, 1986: pp 49–65
110. Flor H, Fydrich T, Turk D C. Efficacy of multidisciplinary pain treatment centres: a meta-analytic review. Pain 1992; 49: 221–230
111. Williams ACdeC, Nicholas M K, Richardson P H et al. Evaluation of a cognitive behavioural programme for rehabilitating patients with chronic pain. Br J General Practice 1993; 43: 513–518
112. Peters J, Large R G, Elkind G. Follow-up results from a randomised controlled trial evaluating in- and outpatient pain management programmes. Pain 1992; 50: 41–50
113. Goodman J E, McGrath P J. The epidemiology of pain in children and adolescents: a review. Pain 1991; 46: 247–264
114. Davis R W. Phantom sensation, phantom pain and stump pain. Arch Phys Med Rehabil 1993; 74: 79–91
115. Steege J F, Stout A L, Somkuti SG. Chronic pelvic pain in women: toward an integrative model. Obstet Gynaecol Surv 1993; 48: 95–110
116. Foster J M G. Chronic perineal pain. Pain Rev 1994; 1: 116–120
117. Van de Kelft E, Van Vyre M. Chronic perineal pain related to sacral meningeal cysts. Neurosurgery 1991; 29: 223–226
118. Boas R A, Schug S A, Acland R H. Perineal pain after rectal amputation; a 5–year follow-up. Pain 1993; 52: 67–70
119. Frank A. Low back pain. BMJ 1993; 306: 901–909
120. Jayson M I V. Mechanisms underlying chronic back pain. BMJ 1994; 309: 681–682
121. Compston J E. The therapeutic use of bisphosphonates. BMJ 1994; 309: 711–715
122. Barnsley L, Lord S, Bogduk N. Whiplash injury. Pain 1994; 58: 283–307
123. Boivie J. Central Pain. In: Wall P D, Melzack R. (eds) Textbook of Pain. 3rd edn. Churchill Livingstone, London, 1994: pp 871– 902
124. Platt O S, Thorington D R. Pain in sickle cell disease: rates and risk factors. N Engl J Med 1991; 325: 11–16
125. O'Neill W M, Sherrard J S. Pain in human immunodeficiency virus disease: a review. Pain 1993; 54: 3–14
126. Wilson A, Hiskie I, Lloyd A et al. Longitudinal study of outcome of chronic fatigue syndrome. BMJ 1994; 308: 756–759
127. Barton N J, Hooper G, Noble J, Steel W M. Occupational causes of disorders in the upper limb. BMJ 1992; 304: 309–311
128. Croft P, Schollum J, Silman A. Population study of tender point counts and pain as evidence of fibromyalgia. BMJ 1994; 309: 696–699
129. Cohen M L, Quinter J L. Fibromyalgia syndrome, a problem of tautology. Lancet 1993; 342: 906–909
130. Rosomoff H L, Fishbain D A, Goldberg M et al. Physical findings in patients with chronic intractable benign pain of the neck and/or back. Pain 1989; 37: 279–287
131. Mendelson G. Compensation and chronic pain. Pain 1992; 48: 121–123
132. Macrae W A, Davies H T O, Crombie I K. Pain: paradigms and treatments. Pain 1992; 49: 289–291

10

Recent developments in septic shock

J–L Vincent

INTRODUCTION

Septic shock remains one of the most common causes of morbidity and mortality amongst critically ill patients. The true incidence of this disease has been difficult to establish, due largely to a lack of consensus in the definition of sepsis and its sequelae. Recently, however, efforts have been made to introduce unambiguous criteria for defining sepsis, sepsis syndrome and septic shock.[1,2] Accordingly, septic shock describes the clinical syndrome corresponding to acute circulatory failure resulting from serious infection. This presents as arterial hypotension (systolic arterial pressure below 90 mmHg or mean arterial pressure below 60 mmHg) associated with altered mental status, changes in organ perfusion and signs of organ failure, such as a reduction in urine output. Sometimes, decreased skin perfusion may be observed. Increased blood lactate levels (>2 mEq/L; >2 mmol/L) reflect alterations in cellular metabolism.

Although typically regarded as a consequence of infection by Gram-negative bacteria, septic shock may also be provoked by Gram-positive organisms and, it is suspected, by fungi, viruses and parasites as well. There is evidence to suggest that the incidence of sepsis and its sequelae is increasing. In US hospitals between 1979 and 1987, the reported incidence of sepsis syndrome increased by 139%, from 73.6 to 175.9 per 100 000 persons discharged.[3] This increased risk of infection is probably related to the technological advances in medical procedures that have been made during the latter half of this century, for example: the aggressive use of catheters and other invasive equipment, the implantation of prosthetic devices and the administration of chemotherapy and immunosuppressive agents. In addition, advances in medical care have offered increased life spans to the elderly and immunodeficient, but these patients remain at increased risk of infection.[1,4]

The pathophysiology of septic shock involves an extremely complex interplay between tissue hypoxia and the host's immune response. In the first few days following the onset of illness, death from septic shock is frequently caused by refractory hypotension with a low systemic vascular resistance. The most frequent cause of death in later stages of the disease is sepsis-induced multiple organ failure (MOF), typical examples being pulmonary failure from adult (or acute) respiratory distress syndrome (ARDS) and renal failure.[4] Therefore, even in those patients for whom resuscitation succeeds in restoring blood pressure, septic shock may still present the risk of subsequent MOF.

Clearly, the successful treatment of septic shock depends on effective responses to both the hypoxic and immunological alterations. The immediate aim must be to sustain organ function through haemodynamic stabilization thus facilitating the definitive treatment, based on the removal of the source of sepsis and the administration of medications directed against the infectious organisms. Advances have been made in two major areas. First, resuscitation regimens have been improved with the aim of augmenting oxygen supply to the cells and thereby preventing tissue hypoxia. Second, new therapeutic options have been offered through a deeper understanding of the immunological alterations provoked by infection. This chapter presents the most recent developments in each of these areas.

RECENT DEVELOPMENTS IN THE CORRECTION OF TISSUE HYPOXIA IN SEPTIC SHOCK

Resuscitation regimens have benefited recently from advances in the understanding of the pathophysiological consequences of septic shock. In particular, attention has focused on the effects of myocardial depression. These advances have resulted in the the development of a step-by-step approach to haemodynamic stabilization.

Pathophysiological consequences

The pathophysiological consequences observed in septic shock are characterized by major alterations in the balance between the demand, extraction and transport of oxygen, the latter being strongly influenced by myocardial depression (Figure 10.1).

Increased oxygen demand

Severe sepsis is characterized by increased oxygen requirements which result from both direct cellular activation and indirect stimulation secondary to the hormonal stress response.[5] Many cytokines and other mediators are involved in this process. Hyperthermia is only one component of this inflammatory reaction, since cellular metabolism remains elevated in the absence of fever.

Altered oxygen extraction

The release of various mediators is also involved in the alteration of vascular tone and blood flow. In particular, the activation of leukocytes, platelets and other cellular elements have been implicated in capillary obstruction,

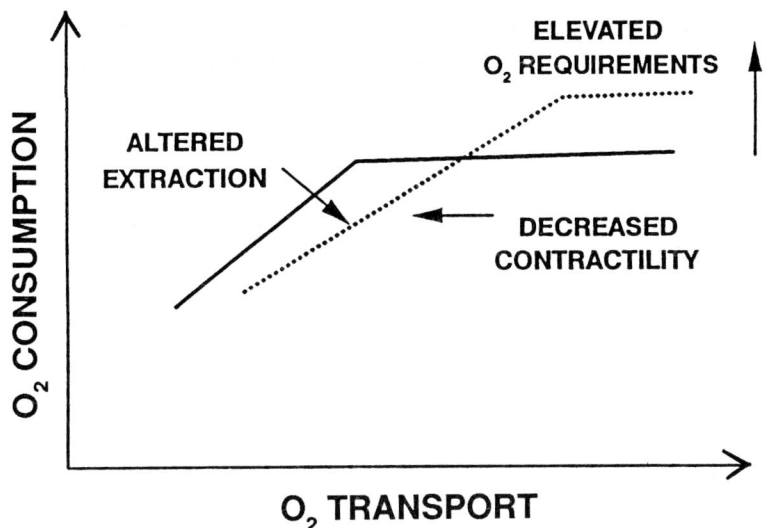

Fig. 10.1   Illustration of the principal haemodynamic alterations in septic shock: elevated oxygen requirements, altered oxygen extraction and decreased myocardial contractility. Solid line denotes normal situation whilst dotted line denotes derrangement.

decreased responsiveness of the arteriolar smooth muscle to adrenergic stimulation, and injury of the endothelial cells resulting in the development of interstitial oedema.[5,6] Maldistribution of blood flow has been implicated in the peripheral vasodilation associated with a reduction in systemic vascular resistance. It appears that the microvascular alterations in septic shock[7] precede the cellular alterations.[8]

Altered oxygen transport

In septic shock, oxygen transport (the product of cardiac output and the arterial oxygen content) is insufficient to satisfy the oxygen demand of the tissues. Two major defects can limit the increase in cardiac output. The first of these defects, reduced venous return, occurs typically in the early stages of severe sepsis. One contributory mechanism is via absolute fluid losses. Such losses are either external (e.g. diarrhoea, burns) or internal (e.g. peritonitis, intestinal sequestration). Another mechanism reducing venous return is the peripheral pooling of blood resulting from peripheral vasodilation. The second defect responsible for reduced cardiac output, myocardial depression, has been the subject of recent research and deserves more detailed discussion.

Myocardial depression

Myocardial contractility can be depressed even when cardiac output is normal or high. This apparent contradiction can be explained by several factors. First, high cardiac output can be attributed to an elevated heart rate but stroke volume might not necessarily be elevated. Second, cardiac output may be maintained by an elevated ventricular preload secondary to generous fluid therapy. Third, and most importantly, the left ventricular ejection is facilitated by the reduced left ventricular preload related to the alterations in peripheral vascular tone (Figure 10.2).

Various experimental studies using animal models have indicated that myocardial contractility is altered early after the administration of endotoxin or live bacteria.[9] Similarly, many clinical studies have indicated that myocardial function, as assessed by the relation between ventricular stroke work and the corresponding filling pressure or the measurement of the ventricular ejection fraction, is depressed early in the course of septic shock.[10,11] Myocardial blood flow is well preserved in animal studies of septic shock. In septic shock patients also, global coronary blood flow is usually well preserved and myocardial lactate production is usually not found.[12] Hence, the presence of myocardial ischaemia does not play a predominant role, at least in the absence of profound hypotension. The release of mediators of sepsis is thought to play a most important role. In various models in vitro and in vivo, tumour necrosis factor α (TNFα) has been shown to reduce myocardial contractility.[13] The role of this and other mediators similarly implicated, including platelet activating factor (PAF), oxygen free radicals and nitric oxide, will be discussed in more detail later.

Since the severity of sepsis is directly related to the degree of release of mediators, it is logical to consider that the severity of myocardial depres-

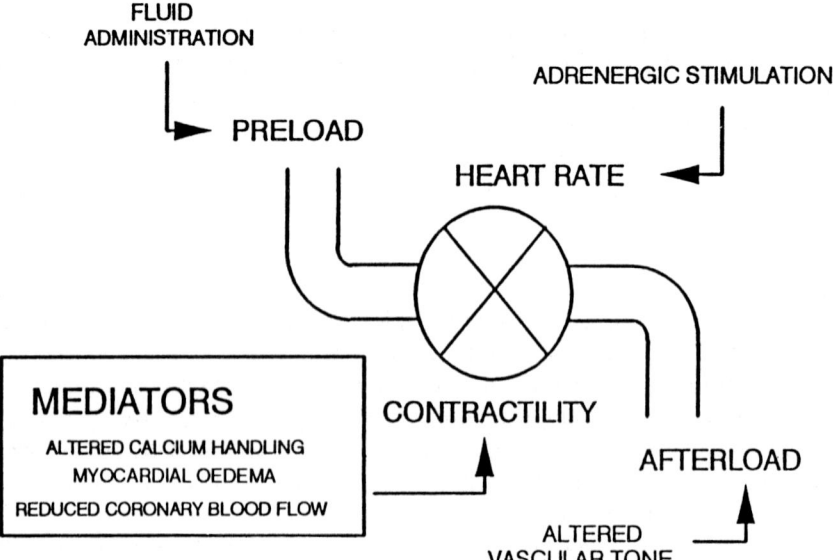

Fig. 10.2 The four parameters that determine cardiac output can be altered in septic shock. Myocardial contractility can be depressed even when cardiac output is normal or high because the three other determinants of cardiac output are altered simultaneously.

sion is directly related to the severity of sepsis. This is indeed supported by a variety of experimental[9,14] and clinical[10,11,15,16] studies. In particular, reduction in myocardial contractility was found to be directly proportional to the amount of endotoxin administered to animals.[14] Several clinical studies also indicated that non-survivors from septic shock have a more severe alteration in ventricular function, as expressed by the relationship between ventricular stroke work and the corresponding cardiac filling pressure.[10,11] Measurements of the right ventricular ejection fraction by the thermodilution technique also revealed that the non-survivors from septic shock have a more severe alteration of their ventricular contractility than the survivors.[15,16] The left ventricular ejection fraction might not show the same pattern, but this is perhaps not too surprising: ventricular function is also influenced by afterload, and the left ventricular afterload is usually more reduced in the non-survivors who also have more severe alterations in systemic vascular tone.[17]

Haemodynamic stabilization

The immediate management of septic shock involves three essential steps based on the underlying defects outlined above: the restoration of blood volume, the restoration of tissue perfusion pressure and the restoration of oxygen delivery. A reduction in oxygen demand can represent another measure to improve the cellular oxygen balance.

First step: restoration of blood volume

The choice of intravenous fluids to be administered in severe infections is still a matter of controversy. The debate is maintained by the lack of proof that one type of fluid is superior to another. This lack of evidence also stresses that many other factors are involved in the survival from severe sepsis. In particular, the appropriate volume of fluid is probably more important than the type of fluid to be administered. It is widely agreed, however, that colloid solutions remain to a larger extent in the intravascular space and therefore the volume required to achieve the same end-points is between two and three times smaller with colloids than with crystalloids.[18] Therefore, the administration of colloids can more rapidly and more easily restore oxygen transport to the cells. In addition, septic patients are prone to develop peripheral oedema, which can contribute to the impairment in cellular oxygenation by increasing the diffusion gradient for oxygen from the capillaries to the cells. A major argument against the use of colloids has been the elevated cost of the natural products. However, the availability of synthetic colloids, benefiting from safe, effective and relatively inexpensive administration, has played down the importance of this cost factor. In addition, recent studies have suggested that hydroxyethylstarch (HES) solutions might reduce the capillary leaks in experimental models of sepsis with associated multiple organ failure.[19]

The volume of fluids required is highly variable. Certainly, the total amount needed to achieve immediate resuscitation cannot be based on the patient's fluid balance. A corollary statement is that the fluid infusion cannot be discontinued on the basis that large amounts of fluids have already been infused. Sometimes massively positive fluid balances are required to restore volume even in the absence of evident fluid losses. A given level of cardiac filling pressure is a better end point, but still hard to define. An optimal level of pulmonary artery balloon-occluded pressure has been found around 12 mmHg[20] in a study of 15 septic patients. However, higher values might be required transiently in some patients.[21] Measurements of ventricular end-diastolic volumes derived from thermodilution measurements of right ventricular ejection fraction may be useful.[22] In any case, fluid administration should be performed in the form of repeated fluid challenges, the effects of which are serially examined by repeated haemodynamic evaluations. Once cardiac output reaches a plateau, fluid challenge should be discontinued, since a further increase in left-sided filling pressures would only increase the risk of pulmonary oedema.

Transfusion of red blood cells must often be added to the fluid management. The optimal range of haematocrit values can be fairly large, so that a haematocrit of 30 to 35% is usually found to be a safe limit.

Second step: restoration of tissue perfusion pressure

The optimal level of perfusion pressure is difficult to define for all acutely ill patients. In most patients, a systolic blood pressure of 90 to 100 mmHg or a mean arterial pressure of 70 to 75 mmHg is acceptable, but these levels are usually higher in elderly patients than in younger patients. In minor cases, fluid administration alone can be sufficient to restore haemodynamic stability. In the majority of cases, however, the administration of a vasopressor is required to increase arterial pressure. Dopamine or noradrenaline should be selected for this purpose. Dopamine is usually chosen first because it can better maintain organ blood flow. If the doses can be maintained relatively low, the renal and the mesenteric circulations may be selectively preserved. Nevertheless, the routine use of so-called 'renal' doses of dopamine has been seriously challenged.[23]

If hypotension persists despite the dopamine administration at doses of 20 to 25 µg/kg/min, noradrenaline should be added to this regimen. Although some clinicians would recommend to taper down the dopamine infusion to less than 2 µg/kg/min, in an attempt to preserve renal perfusion in the presence of the strong noradrenaline-mediated vasoconstriction, the beneficial effect of this therapeutic intervention remains doubtful. It may be more practical to maintain the dopamine dose and to taper down and discontinue the noradrenaline infusion as soon as the clinical situation has improved.

Once a minimal tissue perfusion pressure has been restored, attempts to further increase systemic vascular resistance with vasopressor agents are not likely to be beneficial. The clinical studies which documented the beneficial effects of noradrenaline in patients with severe septic shock, sometimes associated with an improvement in renal function, all included patients with profound hypotension[24-27] but any beneficial effect in less severe hypotension has not been established. Practically, this can result in a further increase in arterial pressure, which is not necessarily beneficial, or limit blood flow and oxygen delivery, which can even be detrimental to the tissues. Vasoconstrictive agents have not been shown clearly to improve the oxygen extraction capabilities in septic shock.[28] Therefore, vasopressor therapy should be based on measurements of arterial pressure rather than systemic vascular resistance.

Third step: restoration of oxygen delivery

Once a minimal tissue perfusion has been restored, attention should focus on the restoration of a sufficient oxygen delivery to the tissues. The maintenance of a haemoglobin saturation in the arterial blood (SaO_2) above 95% is a fundamental goal in the treatment of any type of acute circulatory failure. In severe respiratory failure, this goal might be difficult to achieve but the SaO_2 should, in any case, be maintained above 90%. This implies that the arterial oxygen tension (PaO_2) should be above 8.0 kPa (60 mmHg) at all times. Below this value, the SaO_2 falls sharply according to the curvilinear shape of the oxyhaemoglobin dissociation curve. As mentioned earlier, haematocrit should be maintained above 30%. Once this has been achieved, the restoration of oxygen delivery rapidly turns to the essential question of an appropriate cardiac output.

As shown in Figure 10.1, myocardial depression can limit oxygen supply to the tissues even when cardiac output is normal or elevated. The addition of dobutamine in these conditions has been shown to be effective.[29] Figure 10.3 represents the haemodynamic effects of the addition of a standard dose of 5 µg/kg/min to a standard resuscitation regimen. A dose higher than 5 µg/kg/min may be required. The use of dobutamine should result in an increase in cardiac output but no change in arterial pressure, so that systemic vascular resistance will decline. This again emphasizes that treatment should not be based on calculations of systemic vascular resistance. It is, however, difficult to give recommendations regarding the optimal doses of dobutamine or the level of oxygen delivery that should be provided.

Some investigators have recommended to maintain oxygen delivery (DO_2) at supranormal levels in all patients at risk of complications,[30,31] but this approach is limited by the fact that oxygen demand, which cannot be directly determined, may be influenced by a number of determinants, including body temperature, pain and anxiety, type of respiration, and even bedside procedures. It may be preferable to tailor therapy according to a number of criteria presented in Table 10.1. Obviously, clinical evaluation

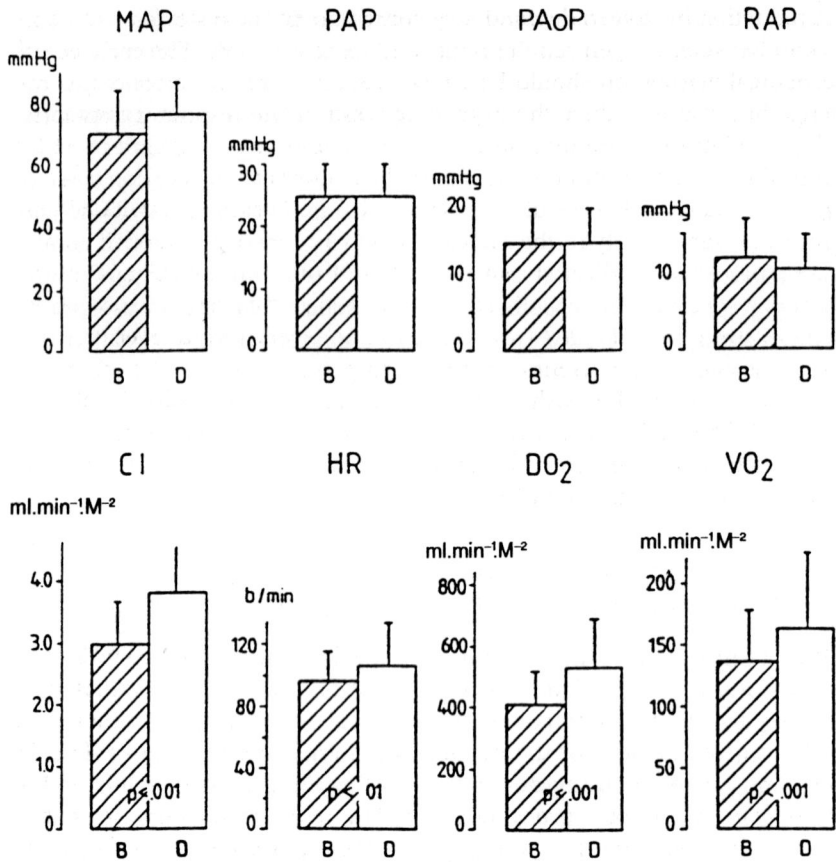

Fig. 10.3   Effects of a dobutamine infusion at a rate of 5 μg/kg/min on mean arterial pressure (MAP), mean pulmonary artery pressure(PAP), pulmonary artery balloon-occluded pressure (PAoP), right atrial pressure (RAP), cardiac index (CI), heart rate (HR), oxygen delivery (DO_2) and oxygen consumption ($\dot{V}O_2$) in 18 patients with septic shock (mean ± SD). Adapted from reference 29.
B = before dobutamine; D = during dobutamine.

remains very important, but this alone may not be sufficient. In particular, the restoration of an adequate blood pressure is not sufficient to establish complete stabilization, since some degree of tissue hypoxia may persist in the absence of hypotension. Monitoring of blood lactate levels is very important, since the presence of tissue hypoxia is very unlikely when the lactate levels are normalized. Repeated determinations of blood lactate concentrations can serve as a useful guide since a rapid resolution of lactic acidosis can reflect the correction of underlying tissue hypoxia.[32] Combination of blood lactate levels and gastric intramucosal pH (pHi) measurements can be useful.[33] In complex cases, the demonstration of oxygen consumption rate versus delivery ($\dot{V}O_2/DO_2$) independency is a valid endpoint, and the use of a cardiac index/oxygen extraction diagram may be useful for this purpose.[34]

A reduction in oxygen demand may contribute to the restoration of equilibrium between oxygen requirements and oxygen supply. The early use of mechanical ventilation should be considered, not only to improve gas exchange but also to reduce the oxygen demand of the respiratory muscles. Hyperventilation is common in severe sepsis and can be exacerbated by the need for compensation of the metabolic acidosis or the development of respiratory failure. The resulting increase in the breathing workload can contribute significantly to the increase in the oxygen demand of the body. Some studies have indicated that the early institution of mechanical ventilation can increase the oxygen availability to the other organs and relieve tissue hypoxia, as indicated by a reduction in blood lactate levels.[35]

Fever is likely to represent a protective mechanism against the infection, so its aggressive combat with antipyretic substances should be critically re-evaluated. The deliberate induction of hypothermia, sometimes used in the past to reduce oxygen demand, has been virtually abandoned, for its problems outweigh the elusive benefits.

RECENT DEVELOPMENTS IN THE UNDERSTANDING OF IMMUNOLOGICAL ALTERATIONS IN SEPTIC SHOCK

Advances in immunology and molecular biology during the past decade reveal that the host's inflammatory response to infection contributes substantially to the development of septic shock.[36-38] Attempts to identify a single central mediator of the disease have been unconvincing to date. It seems more likely that the development of sepsis is related to a complex interplay between many pro- and anti-inflammatory mediators. Recently, many of the mediators involved in the inflammatory and anti-inflammatory responses have been identified, thus facilitating experimentation with a whole new range of therapies. The sepsis cascade is often initiated by the release of endotoxin and/or other microbiological metabolites into the circulation. This prompts the release of TNF-α, interleukin 1 (IL-1), interleukin 6 (IL-6), interleukin 8 (IL-8), and platelet activating factor (PAF) by mononuclear phagocytes and, amongst others, the endothelial cells. After these initial releases, arachidonic acid is metabolized to form leukotrienes, thromboxane A_2 and prostaglandins. IL-1 and IL-6 activate the T-cells to produce further cytokines, including granulocyte colony stimulating factor (GCSF).[39-42]

Whilst it has been possible to identify the network of mediator release (Figure 10.4), identifying the exact role of these mediators is an ongoing and far from simple task. One problem is that these mediators may have beneficial, as well as deleterious effects. In particular, an immunological response is very desirable in response to moderate infection. Another complication is that of varying cellular receptivity to stimuli. Finally, it seems that the mediators of septic shock interact with each other in very complex ways so that even if one pathway of the network is denied, release may be facilitated via another. Indeed, it has been suggested that the number of

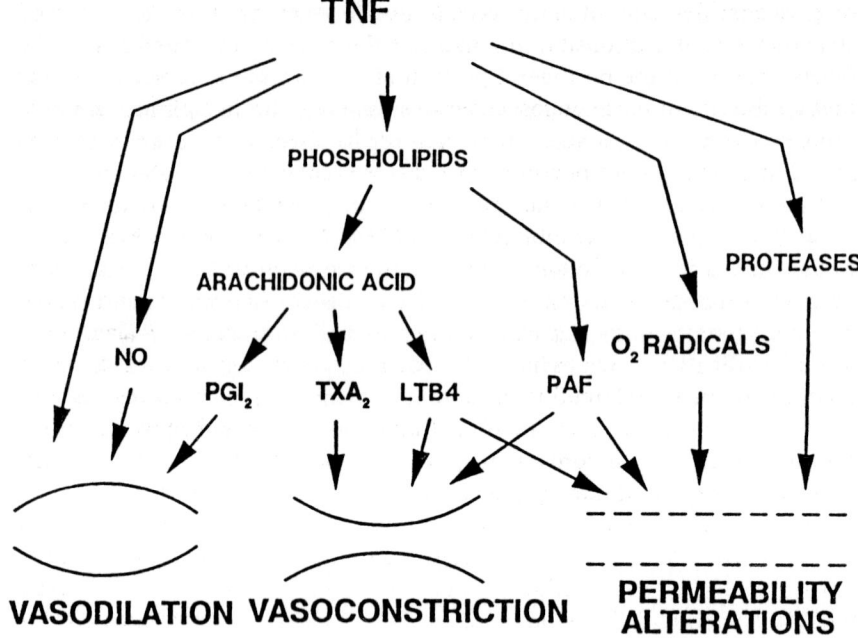

Fig. 10.4 Direct and indirect effects of TNF on the microcirculation.

interactions between mediators may be close to the number of mediators squared.[1] This indicates that a combination therapy, rather than blocking a single mediator, is most likely to offer an effective defence against septic shock.

Having once admitted that the mediators of septic shock are involved in such complex interactions, it may seem artificial to attempt to discuss their roles individually. Nevertheless, the 'key players' in septic shock are presented here, in turn, with the hope of elucidating, as far as possible, the various therapeutic options available.

Endotoxins

Endotoxins occur primarily as lipopolysaccharide (LPS) components of the outer membrane of Gram-negative bacteria[43] and are an extremely potent trigger of the network of mediators and the complement cascade. It is very likely that the endotoxin-invoked inflammatory response is an important weapon in the host's initial defence against infection. However, it is widely believed that persistent or repetitive inflammatory provocation may lead to an 'anarchic' situation, in which the body can no longer control its own inflammatory response.[1] This results in endothelial damage, interstitial oedema and altered organ function. Under these circumstances, the risk of MOF is high.

The endotoxin molecule consists of an outer layer of structurally and antigenically diverse oligosaccharides and a core of similarly structured oligosaccharides. Bound to this core is lipid A which has a highly conserved structure and is responsible for most of the toxicity of endotoxin.[44] The diverse nature of the peripheral portion of the endotoxin molecule means that antibodies to these oligosaccharides have only limited clinical applications. However, greater scope for treatment has been offered by antibodies raised against the core portion since this is similar in all endotoxins.

Two monoclonal antibodies directed at core LPS and lipid A have been developed: E5, a murine monoclonal IgM antibody and HA–1A, a human monoclonal antibody. Following encouraging animal studies,[45,46] there have been several large prospective, randomized, placebo-controlled clinical trials recently of both E5 and HA–1A. The first E5 trial was an evaluation of 468 patients, 316 of whom had a documented Gram-negative infection. In a retrospectively identified subgroup of 137 patients with Gram-negative infection but not refractory shock, E5 improved survival.[47] However, these findings could not be confirmed in a subsequent trial with 847 patients, 530 of whom had Gram-negative infection without refractory shock although a reduced incidence of organ failure was suggested. A third trial is underway to confirm whether E5 may indeed protect against organ failure. An HA–1A trial was conducted similarly to that with E5, but this time with 543 patients.[48] This study indicated that HA–1A could reduce 28–day all-cause mortality and hence was largely responsible for the clinical approval of the treatment in Europe. However, it was suggested later that the protocol of the trial was flawed, and the US Food and Drug Administration demanded a second clinical trial to evaluate HA–1A in the treatment of Gram-negative sepsis.[49] An interim report of this so-called CHESS trial suggested increased mortality in patients without Gram-negative infection and HA–1A was eventually withdrawn from the European market by its manufacturer. These results seem to agree with a canine model of septic shock in which a significantly reduced 28-day survival was observed in those dogs treated with HA–1A, apparently due to deleterious effects on cardiac performance.[50]

Another anti-endotoxin approach is the possibility of using the naturally occurring molecule known as bactericidal permeability-increasing protein (BPI). This occurs in the polymorphonuclear leukocytes and, although not an antibody, binds very strongly with lipid A to inhibit the toxicity of endotoxin. Recombinant BPI has been shown to protect against lethal doses of endotoxin in mice and rats.[51] Studies in humans are being planned.

Finally, it may be possible to protect against lipid A via prophylaxis. It has been found that some types of natural lipid A and synthetic lipid A analogues have low or even no toxicity. This has led to the development of lipid A analogues that can block the toxic effects of endotoxin.[52]

Tumour necrosis factor α

Much attention has been focussed on one of the cytokines, TNF-alpha, since it has several characteristics consistent with being a central mediator of septic shock:

- High blood levels of TNF-alpha are found in those patients with a high probability of death or organ failure.[53-56]
- Administration of TNF in animals leads to septic shock and organ failure.[57] Administration of TNF in volunteers leads to similar effects as those associated with endotoxin infection.[58,59]
- Administration of TNF antibodies in animals can protect against the administration of endotoxin and live bacteria.[38,60,61]

TNF is also incriminated in myocardial depression via several mechanisms, including the development of myocardial oedema, alterations in the myocardial cell membrane or in the contractile apparatus.[9]

Clinical studies are currently concentrating on the effect of blocking TNF-alpha with antibodies in septic shock patients. An initial trial with a murine antibody revealed that whilst there may be beneficial effects for those patients with shock, blocking TNF-α has no beneficial effect on those without septic shock. If anti-TNF-α antibodies are going to provide positive results, it is likely that these will be most apparent in the early stages of infection. In particular, TNF-α antibodies could help to increase ventricular stroke work[62] in response to myocardial depression, as discussed previously.

Research is also being undertaken in the field of naturally soluble receptors to TNF-α. However, a recent study presented worrying results. In a phase II blind, randomized trial, 141 patients with sepsis syndrome received either a placebo or one of three doses of a recombinant human dimeric TNF-α receptor. In the low dose (0.15 mg/kg) and placebo groups, 28–day mortality was found to be the same (30%). Worse outcomes were observed in patients who received medium (0.45 mg/kg, 48%) and high (1.5 mg/kg, 53%) doses. These results raise serious concerns about the potential harmful consequences of anticytokine therapies in sepsis and septic shock patients. A plausible explanation is that blocking TNF-α too avidly or for too long may produce unwanted effects.

Interleukin 1

In common with TNF-α, IL-1 has been associated with a central role in the mediation of septic shock.[36,63-65] Circulating levels of IL-1 increase according to the severity of disease.[54,55] It is probable that the toxic effects of IL-1 are slightly less severe than those of TNF-α. However, when IL-1 and TNF-α are administered in combination, the former has been found to increase the toxicity of the latter.[66]

In animals, interleukin 1 receptor antagonist (IL-1 ra) demonstrated protection against some modes of infection.[36,63-65] Recent clinical trials have studied the effects of IL-1 ra. Following the encouraging results of a phase II trial,[67] the findings of a phase III trial of IL-1 ra were recently disclosed.[68] Nine hundred and one patients with sepsis syndrome and septic shock were included in a randomized, double-blind, placebo-controlled, multicentre clinical trial. Although survival rate was not significantly improved by administration of IL-1 ra, retrospective risk assessment of each patient using a validated scoring system suggested that IL-1 ra may be beneficial in patients with severe sepsis.[69] Unfortunately, a complementary study was recently discontinued due to an interim analysis which showed no beneficial results.

Interleukin 6

IL-6 is expressed as part of the inflammatory response mediated by IL-1 and TNF-α. It in turn mediates the metabolic response of the liver but has little haemodynamic effect.[70] Recent indications are that IL-6 may have anti-inflammatory properties and that therapeutic trials of anti-IL-6 agents would be unproductive.

Interleukin 8

IL-8 is another cytokine provoked by TNF-α and IL-1. It is responsible for the activation of leukocytes. Since IL-8 alone cannot explain most of the alterations observed in septic shock, it is unlikely that anti-IL-8 agents will present significant therapeutic advantages.

Interleukin 10

IL-10 is a cytokine with anti-inflammatory properties. In particular, IL-10 reduces the release of TNF-α following experimental endotoxin challenge and has been associated with increased survival under these conditions.[71] The possible role of IL-10 as a protective cytokine in septic shock has been discussed recently[72] and clinical trials are being considered.

Adhesion molecules

Cytokines such as TNF-α and IL-1 induce the expression of adhesion molecules which mediate the interactions between endothelial cells and polymorphonuclear cells (PMN) and play an important role in the circulatory system. Adhesion molecules occur in three different forms:

The immunoglobulin superfamily

This includes the antigen-specific receptors of the T and B lymphocytes and the intercellular adhesion molecule 1 (ICAM 1). The induction of ICAM 1 is sustained in sepsis.

The selectin family

These adhesion molecules interact with neutrophils and lymphocytes. An important selectin in the context of septic shock is the endothelial cell leukocyte adhesion molecule 1 (ELAM 1) which is induced by TNF-α and IL-1 up to 8 hours after endotoxin administration.

The integrins family

This interferes with leukocyte activation, platelet adhesion and cell migration. Members include several leukocyte membrane proteins such as the CD 11–CD 18 glycoprotein complex which regulates important leukocyte functions.

Several antibodies to adhesion molecules have resulted from recent biotechnological developments. Monoclonal antibodies to the CD 11 B-18 complex have been administered in animals in an attempt to reduce the leukocyte mediated injury during hemorrhagic shock in primates[73] and rabbits.[74] The administration of these antibodies has been shown to reduce organ damage and to attenuate myocardial injury in dogs.[75] Moreover, these antibodies have also been found to be protective in some models of sepsis. An antibody to CD 11B increased PaO_2 and improved survival rate in dogs given TNF-α,[76] whilst in a pig model of sepsis, induced by live *Pseudomonas*, these antibodies attenuated neutropenia and reduced the alveolar capillary membrane damage.[77] Nevertheless, some studies suggest that these antibodies may present the risk of increased infection. In rabbits, an antibody to CD 18 did not increase the septic response but increased the size of abscess due to *Staphylococcus*.[78] Recently, a murine monoclonal antibody to CD 18 was administered in a model of intraperitoneal sepsis in conscious dogs.[79] Although the differences were not statistically significant, the survival time was shorter in the animals treated with this antibody compared with those treated with antibiotics and intravenous fluids. The antibody-treated animals showed signs of worse cardiovascular function, more severe lactic acidosis, greater increase in endotoxin levels and lower glucose concentration. These elements, amongst others, suggested that this antibody aggravated rather than attenuated the signs of sepsis in those animals. This could be explained by a reduced accumulation of polynuclear neutrophils at the site of infection. In this context, it is important to note that, owing to a genetic defect, some humans do not express adhesion molecules, and these individuals are more prone to develop severe infections.[80] In vitro studies indicated that neutrophils deficient in the CD 11–18 complex or treated with an antibody to this complex, have an impaired phagocytic ability in response to bacteria and endotoxin.[81,82]

Arachidonic acid metabolites

Arachidonic acid metabolites are released by leukocytes, macrophages and pulmonary endothelial cells, via the cyclo-oxygenase and lipoxygenase pathways. As with many of the mediators already discussed, these metabolites have been implicated in both beneficial and deleterious effects associated with the host's response to septic shock. Therapeutic options include inhibition of one or both of the metabolic pathways, as well as enhancing the beneficial effects and reducing the deleterious effects of some of the metabolic products.

Ibuprofen, indomethacin, meclofenamic acid and other such cyclo-oxygenase inhibitors have been shown to reduce sepsis-induced lung damage in various experimental models[83,84] by assisting in the reduction of pulmonary hypertension, improving lung compliance and also increasing arterial oxygen tension. In goats with *E. coli* sepsis, ibuprofen could reduce total fluid filtration, but did not prevent the permeability defect. A large clinical trial of ibuprofen is currently underway with sepsis syndrome patients in North America.

Prostaglandins, which are produced via the cyclo-oxygenase pathway, could play a protective role in septic shock although studies on the administration of prostaglandin E_1 (PGE_1) have yielded conflicting results. PGE_1 has been reported to have protective effects in several models of severe sepsis and has been shown to improve oxygen extraction capabilities.[85] Patients with ARDS may be protected by PGE_1 but, despite some encouraging studies, this remains to be confirmed. A large multicentre, placebo-controlled study could not demonstrate a beneficial effect of PGE_1 in ARDS.[86]

Thromboxane, another cyclo-oxygenase product, induces potent pulmonary vasoconstriction, bronchoconstriction, and platelet aggregation. Experimentally, thromboxane inhibition can reverse these effects but does not influence the permeability abnormalities.[84] Clinically, the effects of thromboxane inhibitors like dazoxiben have not been encouraging.[87]

The lipoxygenase pathway leads to the formation of leukotrienes which have been implicated in ARDS.[88] Leukotrienes can also participate in the development of pulmonary vasoconstriction, bronchoconstriction, permeability alterations and, possibly, coronary constriction and myocardial depression. Inhibiting lipoxygenase in endotoxic sheep resulted in less marked alterations in haemodynamics, gas exchange and fluid extravasation.[89]

Inhibitors of the phospholipase A_2 such as mepacrine, and other interventions that can inhibit both the cyclo-oxygenase and the lipoxygenase pathways have been attempted with positive effects.

Platelet activating factor

The phosholipid mediator, PAF, can be produced by cytokines as well as macrophages, neutrophils, eosinophils, endothelial cells, and platelets.[90–93] Elevated levels of PAF have been detected in endotoxin-induced hypotension and endotoxin-induced lung injury in rats.[94,95] The effects of TNF-α have been shown to be markedly reduced in the absence of PAF.[96,97]

PAF can alter the vascular tone and also exert a negative inotropic effect on the heart which may contribute to a decrease in arterial blood pressure.

It has also been implicated in pulmonary hypertension.[94] Other major effects of PAF include an increase in microvascular permeability thus promoting microvascular fluid loss, and platelet aggregation causing thrombosis. Recently, the results of a randomized clinical trial of a PAF antagonist were reported.[98] Two hundred and sixty-two patients suffering from severe sepsis received either placebo or PAF antagonist. In a subset of patients with documented Gram-negative sepsis, mortality was found to decrease by 42%. Other trials with PAF antagonists are under way or in preparation.

Oxygen free radicals

Oxygen free radicals are highly reactive agents which may be produced by the enzymes of activated granulocytes and macrophages. Close contact with oxygen free radicals causes alterations in the permeability of the vascular endothelium and alveolar epithelium. In particular H_2O_2 and hydroxyl radicals are responsible for endothelial damage and oedema.[99,100] Oxygen free radicals have been implicated in myocardial depression. Another effect is the inactivation of the alpha-1–proteinase inhibitor thus promoting the destructive action of liberated proteinases.[101] The augmentation of vascular permeability by oxygen free radicals implicates them in the mediation of ARDS.[102]

A number of therapeutic options are associated with the blocking of oxygen free radicals. The lung is protected against oxygen toxicity, endotoxin and other forms of injury by the free radical scavengers superoxide dismutase and catalase.[103] Nonenzymatic scavengers such as vitamins C and E, N-acetylcysteine or dimethylthiourea have also demonstrated protective effects.[104,105] Endothelial cells are protected against phorbal ester-stimulated leukocytes in vitro by dapsone, a drug that can reduce the generation of toxic oxygen radicals.[106] Iron-chelating agents, such as desferrioxamine, which inhibit the catalysis of hydroxyl radicals, have also been tried with some success.[107] Clinical trials with N-acetylcysteine are presently underway. N-acetylcysteine is particularly attractive because it can augment the O_2 extraction capabilities in septic shock and improve haemodynamic performance.[108,109]

Nitric oxide

The constitutional synthase of nitric oxide (NO) via the endothelial cells is calcium dependent and has an important role in physiological vasodilation and neurotransmission. Mediators of septic shock such as TNF-α and endotoxin can, however, induce calcium independent synthase of NO[110] which is thought to be responsible for the decrease in arterial pressure associated with septic shock[111] (Figure 10.5). NO has also been implicated in myocardial depression[112] and is thought to have direct cytotoxic effects leading to tissue injury and organ failure.[113,114]

There is a possibility that NO synthesis inhibitors may increase survival rates in septic shock by increasing mean arterial pressure and reducing cytotoxic damage. However, experimental data are controversial. In a recent study, N-ω amino-L-arginine (L-NAA) was administered continuously for 22 hours to endotoxic and healthy dogs in two doses (1 mg/kg per hour and 10 mg/kg per hour). Whilst cardiac delivery, oxygen delivery and oxygen consumption indices were reduced, systemic vascular resistance was increased.[115] In the same study, doses which did not significantly increase arterial pressure decreased survival time and high doses given to healthy dogs caused seizure. In an attempt to provide more conclusive data, a study was conducted using monomethyl-L-arginine (L-NMMA), another NO synthase inhibitor. Previous animal studies have shown that L-NMMA can increase vascular tone after the administration of LPS[116] or endotoxin.[117] Furthermore it has been observed that a dose of 10 mg/kg of L-NMMA in endotoxic rats could prevent the decrease in blood pressure and hence increase survival whilst a higher dose (300 mg/kg), which also increased blood pressure, increased mortality rate.[118,119] In this most recent study,[120] L-NMMA was administered in doses of 1, 2, 4 and 10 mg/kg per hour. The findings were not encouraging: results similar to those of the previous L-NAA trials were observed together with increased lactic acidosis, hepatic toxicity and, at the highest dose, increased mortality.

It seems that, in addition to the dosage, the timing of NO inhibition plays an important role. Clearly, L-NMMA increases arterial pressure in normal individuals and immediately after endotoxin administration when

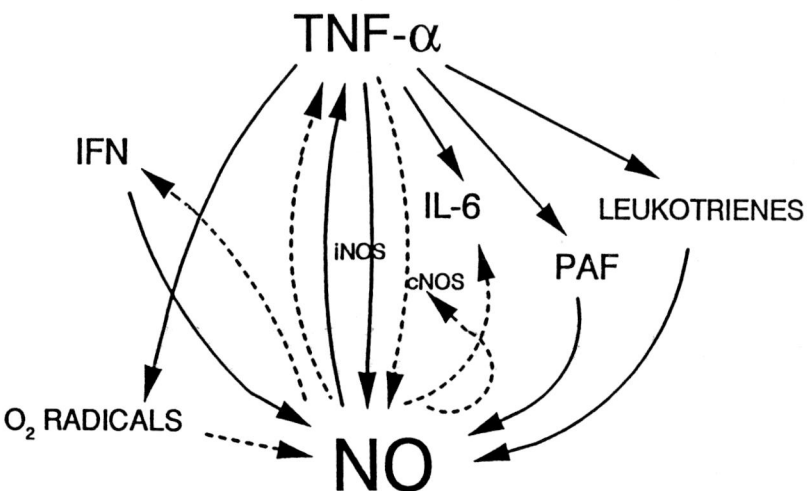

Fig. 10.5   The complex interrelations between TNF-α and NO. Stimulating effects are represented by continuous lines and inhibitory effects by interrupted lines.
iNOS denotes nitric oxide synthase inhibitor.
cNOS denotes cyclic nitric oxide synthase.

the NO synthase has had no time to be induced.[121] Recent studies suggest that blocking NO very early, before the induced synthase is expressed, may be harmful whilst later intervention may be beneficial. Evidence suggests, therefore, that NO inhibition may have both beneficial and deleterious effects depending on both the dosage and the timing of administration.

There have been preliminary reports on the administration of L-NMMA in human beings.[122] These suggested that a blockade of the NO synthase may increase blood pressure but not cardiac output. Studies looking at effects on morbidity and mortality are under way.

Another way to interfere with the haemodynamic effects of NO may be the administration of methylene blue. Methylene blue is an inhibitor of guanylate cyclase which can therefore block the vasodilating effects of NO on the vascular smooth muscle while preserving its neurotransmissive and antimicrobal activity. Recently, a study including 14 patients with severe septic shock, requiring adrenergic therapy, observed that methylene blue at a dose of 2 mg/kg could substantially increase mean arterial pressure. However, this intervention did not significantly affect cardiac output, oxygen delivery or oxygen consumption. A reduction in blood lactate levels was observed, but this could be due to the reducing effects of methylene blue.[123]

Corticosteroids

Corticosteroids are potent anti-inflammatory agents acting chiefly through the inhibition of the phospholipase A2, the enzyme responsible for the generation of arachidonic acid metabolites and PAF. Corticosteroids also inhibit the activation of the complement cascade and the synthesis of TNF-α and IL-1[124] and have been shown to inhibit the induction of NO synthase by endotoxin.[125] The latter mechanism may explain why corti-costeroids have been found effective when administered before or very early during the septic challenge and why this efficacy was lost when the administration took place later as a therapeutic intervention.

Some experimental studies documented a protective effect of steroids in various models of lung injury, but some others could not.[126] Large double-blind, randomized, multicentric studies could not demonstrate any beneficial effect of corticosteroid administration in ARDS patients.[127–129] Steroid therapy could even have adverse effects in surgical patients at risk of ARDS.[130]

Granulocyte colony-stimulating factor (GCSF)

GCSF is a potent stimulator of the neutrophilic immunological response.[131,132] Whereas many of the treatments so far discussed have looked at ways of blocking this response, GCSF treatment aims to increase it. An animal study evaluated the administration of GCSF or placebo 9 days before and

3 days after infection.[133] Before infection, neutrophil count was increased by a factor of up to six. After infection, the therapy was associated with prolonged survival times, improved arterial blood pressure and improved cardiac function. Clearance of endotoxin was also noted.

In septic shock patients, stimulating an already anarchic immune response is probably unwise. However, this treatment may prove successful in fortifying a patient once a stable condition has been restored.

CONCLUSION

Haemodynamic management of septic shock should be based first on early and effective volume replacement, second on restoration of a minimal tissue perfusion and finally on an adequate oxygen supply to the cells. In addition, it has been found that an inotropic support is often needed to counteract the effects of the myocardial depression associated with severe sepsis. Lastly, a reduction in the oxygen needs of the cells can contribute to improve the balance between oxygen demand and oxygen supply. Improved resuscitation techniques can reduce not only morbidity but also early mortality in septic shock.

Evidently, the results of immunological therapies in septic shock to date remain inconclusive, despite much of the recent progress in identifying and understanding the processes of mediation of the disease. It is clear that there are no clinically acceptable therapeutic implications at the present time, but this is no reason to be pessimistic. Immunological therapies are still in their infancy and need time to develop. The trials already performed have helped to deepen the understanding of the machinery involved. One of the major tasks remains to identify the patients who may benefit from treatment. This is undoubtedly the underlying problem at present and represents the major determinant of outcome in the treatment of septic shock.

KEY POINTS FOR CLINICAL PRACTICE

- Control of infection
    Antibiotic therapy
    Control of the source if needed
    (surgical drainage, percutaneous drainage, etc.)
- Haemodynamic resuscitation
    Fluid therapy
    (under control of cardiac filling pressures)
    Vasopressor therapy
    (initial drug is dopamine, but noradrenaline may be also required)
    Inotropic therapy to increase oxygen delivery to the tissues
    (dobutamine is the preferred agent)
- Immunotherapy
    Only experimental (nothing available today)

REFERENCES

1. Bone R C. The pathogenesis of sepsis. Ann Intern Med 1991; 115: 457–469
2. Vincent J L. Sepsis and septic shock: Update on definitions. In: Eyrich K, Sprung C and Reinhart K (eds) Update in Intensive Care and Emergency Medicine. Springer Verlag, Berlin, 1994; pp 3–15
3. Increase in National Hospital Discharge Survey rates for septicemia – United States, 1979–1987. MMWR Morb Mortal Wkly Rep 1990; 39: 31–34
4. Vincent J L. Diagnostic and medical management/supportive care of patients with Gram negative bacteremia and septic shock. Infect Dis Clin North Am 1991; 5: 807–816
5. Merrill G F, Rosolowsky M. Effect of dichloroacetate sodium on the lactacidemia of experimental endotoxin shock. Circ Shock 1980; 7: 13–21
6. Rackow E C, Astiz M E, Weil M H. Cellular oxygen metabolism during sepsis and shock. The relationship of oxygen consumption to oxygen delivery. JAMA 1988; 259: 1989–1993
7. Geller E R, Jankauskas S, Kirkpatrick J. Mitochondrial death in sepsis: a failed concept. J Surg Res 1986; 40: 514–519
8. Mela L, Bacalzo L V, Miller L D. Defective oxidative metabolism of rat mitochondria in hemorrhagic and endotoxin shock. Am J Physiol 1971; 220: 571–580
9. Abel F L. Myocardial function in sepsis and endotoxin shock. Am J Physiol 1989; 257: R1265–R1281
10. D'Orio V, Mendes P, Saad G, Marcelle R. Accuracy in early prediction of prognosis of patients with septic shock by analysis of simple indices: prospective study. Crit Care Med 1990; 18: 1339–1345
11. Vincent J L, Weil M H, Puri V, Carlson R W. Circulatory shock associated with purulent peritonitis. Am J Surg 1981; 142: 262–270
12. Cunnion R E, Schaer G L, Parker M M et al. The coronary circulation in human septic shock. Circulation 1986; 73: 637–644
13. Natanson C, Eichenholz P W, Danner R L et al. Endotoxin and tumor necrosis factor challenges in dogs simulate the cardiovascular profile of human septic shock. J Exp Med 1989; 169: 823–832
14. McDonough K W, Brumfield B A, Lang C H. In vitro myocardial performance after lethal and nonlethal doses of endotoxin. Am J Physiol 1986; 250: H240–H246
15. Vincent J L, Frank R N, Contempre B, Kahn R J. Right ventricular dysfunction in septic shock: Assessment by measurements of right ventricular ejection fraction using the thermodilution technique. Acta Anaesthesiol Scand 1989; 33: 34–38
16. Vincent J L, Gris P, Coffernils M et al. Myocardial depression characterizes the fatal course of septic shock. Surgery 1992; 111: 660–667
17. Parker M M, Suffredini A F, Natanson C et al. Responses of left ventricular function in survivors and nonsurvivors of septic shock. J Crit Care 1989; 4: 19–25
18. Vincent J L. Fluids for resuscitation. Br J Anaesth 1991; 67: 185–193
19. Vincent J L. Plugging the leaks? New insights into synthetic colloids. Crit Care Med 1991; 19: 316–318
20. Packman M I, Rackow L C. Optimum left heart filling pressures during fluid resuscitation of patients with hypovolemic and septic shock. Crit Care Med 1983; 11: 165–169
21. Azimi G, Vincent J L. Ultimate survival from septic shock. Resuscitation 1986; 14: 245–253
22. Reuse C, Vincent J L, Pinsky M R. Measurements of right ventricular volumes during fluid challenge. Chest 1990; 98: 1450–1454
23. Vincent J L. Renal effects of dopamine: may our dream ever come true? (Editorial). Crit Care Med 1994; 22: 5–6
24. Desjars P H, Pinaud M, Bugnon D, Tasseau F. Norepinephrine therapy has no deleterious renal effects in human septic shock. Crit Care Med 1989; 17: 426–429
25. Fukuoka T, Nishimura M, Imanaka H et al. Effects of norepinephrine on renal function in septic patients with normal and elevated serum lactate levels. Crit Care Med 1989; 17: 1104–1107

26. Martin C, Saux P, Albanese J et al. Right ventricular function during positive end-expiratory pressure: thermodilution evaluation and clinical application. Chest 1987; 92: 999–1004
27. Meadows D, Edwards J D, Wilkins R G, Nightingale P. Reversal of intractable septic shock with norepinephrine therapy. Crit Care Med 1988; 16: 663–666
28. Bakker J, Vincent J L. The effects of norepinephrine and dobutamine on oxygen transport and consumption in a dog model of endotoxic shock. Crit Care Med 1993; 21: 425–432
29. Vincent J L, Roman A, Kahn R J. Dobutamine administration in septic shock: Addition to a standard protocol. Crit Care Med 1990; 18: 689–693
30. Shoemaker W C, Appel P L, Kram H B et al. Prospective trial of supranormal values of survivors as therapeutic goals in high-risk surgical patients. Chest 1988; 94: 1176–1186
31. Tuchschmidt J, Fried J, Astiz M, Rackow E. Elevation of cardiac output and oxygen delivery improves outcome in septic shock. Chest 1992; 102: 216–220
32. Vincent J L, Dufaye P, Berre J et al. Serial lactate determinations during circulatory shock. Crit Care Med 1983; 11: 449–451
33. Friedman G, Berlot G, Kahn R J, Vincent J L. Combined measurements of blood lactate levels and gastric intramucosal pH in patients with severe sepsis. Crit Care Med 1995; (in press)
34. Vincent J L, Silance P G, De Backer D. The cardiac index/oxygen extraction diagram to assess hemodynamic status. In: Vincent J L (ed) Yearbook in Intensive Care and Emergency Medicine – 1994. Springer Verlag, Berlin, 1994; pp 144–151
35. Aubier M, Syllie G, Mozes R, Roussos Ch. Respiratory muscle contributing to lactic acidosis in low cardiac output. Am Rev Respir Dis 1982; 126: 648–652
36. Dinarello C A, Wolff S M. The role of interleukin-1 in disease. N Engl J Med 1982; 328: 106–113
37. Nathan C, Sporn M. Cytokines in context. J Cell Biol 1991; 113: 981–986
38. Tracey K J, Fong Y, Hesse D. Anticachectin/TNF alpha monoclonal antibodies prevent septic shock during lethal bacteraemia. Nature 1987; 330: 662–664
39. Johnston R B J. Current concepts: immunology. Monocytes and macrophages. N Engl J Med 1988; 318: 747–752
40. Tracey K J, Vlassara H, Cerami A. Cachectin/tumour necrosis factor. Lancet i: 1989; 1122–1126
41. Jacobs R F, Tabor D R. Immune cellular interactions during sepsis and septic injury. Crit Care Clin 1989; 5: 9–26
42. Kuhweide R, Van Damme J, Ceuppens J L. Tumor necrosis factor-alpha and interleukin 6 synergistically induce T cell growth. Eur J Immunol 1990; 20: 1019–1025
43. Westphal O, Jann K, Himmelspach K. Chemistry and immunochemistry of bacterial lipopolysaccharides as cell wall antigens and endotoxins. Prog Allergy 1983; 33: 9–39
44. Glauser M P, Heumann D, Baumgartner J D, Cohen J. Pathogenesis and potential strategies for prevention and treatment of septic shock: an update. Clin Inf Dis 1994; 18: S205–S216
45. Young L S, Gascon R, Alam S, Bermuder L M. Monoclonal antibodies for treatment of Gram negative infections. Rev Infect Dis 1989; 11: S1564–S1571
46. Teng N N, Kaplan H S, Hebert J M et al. Protection against Gram negative bacteremia and endotoxemia with human monoclonal IgM antibodies. Proc Natl Acad Sci USA 1985; 82: 1790–1794
47. Greenman R L, Schein R M H, Martin M A et al. A controlled clinical trial of E5 murine monoclonal IgM antibody to endotoxin in the treatment of Gram negative sepsis. JAMA 1991; 266: 1097–1102
48. Ziegler E J, Fisher C J, Sprung C L et al. Treatment of gram-negative bacteremia and septic shock with HA-1A human monoclonal antibody against endotoxin. N Engl J Med 1991; 324: 429–436
49. McCloskey R V, Straube R C, Sanders C et al. Chess Trial Study Group. Treatment of septic shock with human monoclonal antibody HA-1A. A randomized, double-blind, placebo-controlled trial. Ann Intern Med 1994; 121: 1–5

50. Quezado Z M, Natanson C, Alling D W et al. A controlled trial of HA-1A in a canine model of gram-negative septic shock. JAMA 1993; 269: 2221–2227
51. Kohn F R, Ammons W S, Horwitz A et al. Protective effect of a recombinant amino-terminal fragment of bactericidal/permeability-increasing protein in experimental endotoxemia. J Infect Dis 1993; 168: 1307–1310
52. Stutz P, Liehl E. Lipid A analogs aimed at preventing the detrimental effects of endotoxin. Infect Dis Clin North Am 1991; 5: 847–873
53. Waage A, Brandtzae G P, Halstensen A et al. The complex pattern of cytokines in serum from patients with meningococcal septic shock. J Exp Med 1989; 189: 333–338
54. Waage A, Halstensen A, Shalaby R et al. Local production of tumor necrosis factor alpha, interleukin 1, and interleukin 6 in meningococcal meningitis. Relation to the inflammatory response. J Exp Med 1989; 170: 1859–1867
55. Calandra T, Baumgartner J D, Grau D G et al. Prognostic values of tumor necrosis factor/cachectin, interleukin-1, interferon-alpha, and interferon-gamma in the serum of patients with septic shock. J Infect Dis 1990; 161: 982–987
56. Pinsky M R, Vincent J L, Deviere J et al. Serum cytokine levels in human septic shock: Relation to multiple-systems organ failure and mortality. Chest 1993; 103: 565–575
57. Stephens K E, Ishizaka A, Larrick J W, Raffin T A. Tumor necrosis factor causes increased pulmonary permeability and edema. Am Rev Respir Dis 1989; 137: 1364–1370
58. Van der Poll T, van Deventer S J H, ten Cate H et al. Tumor Necrosis Factor is involved in the appearance of Interleukin-1 receptor antagonist in endotoxemia. J Infect Dis 1994; 169: 665–667
59. Van der Poll T, Buller H R, ten Cate H et al. Activation of coagulation after administration of tumor necrosis factor to normal subjects. N Engl J Med 1990; 3222: 1622–1626
60. Beutler B, Milsark I W, Cerami A. Passive immunization against cachectin/TNF protects mice from lethal effect of endotoxin. Science 1985; 229: 869–871
61. Opal S M, Cross A S, Kelly N M et al. Efficacy of a monoclonal antibody directed against tumor necrosis factor in protecting neutropenic rats from lethal infection with *Pseudomonas aeruginosa.* J Infect Dis 1990; 161: 1148–1152
62. Vincent J L, Bakker J, Marécaux G et al. Anti-TNF antibodies administration increases myocardial contractility in septic shock patients. Chest 1992; 101: 810–815
63. McIntyre K W, Stepan G J, Kolinsky K D et al. Inhibition of interleukin 1 (IL-1) binding and bioactivity in vitro and modulation of acute inflammation in vivo by IL-1 receptor antagonist and anti-IL-1 receptor monoclonal antibody. J Exp Med 1991; 173: 931–939
64. Wakabayashi G, Gelfand J A, Burke J F et al. A specific receptor antagonist for interleukin 1 prevents *Escherichia coli*-induced shock in rabbits. FASEB J 1991; 5: 338–343
65. Alexander H R, Doherty G M, Buresh C M et al. A recombinant human receptor antagonist to interleukin 1 improves survival after lethal endotoxemia in mice. J Exp Med 1991; 173: 1029–1032
66. Waage A, Espevik T. Interleukin-1 potentiates the lethal effect of tumor necrosis factor alpha/cachectin in mice. J Exp Med 1988; 167: 1987–1992
67. Fisher C J, Slotman G J, Opal S M et al. IL-1RA Sepsis Syndrome Study Group. Initial evaluation of human recombinant interleukin-1 receptor antagonist in the treatment of sepsis syndrome: a randomized, open-label, placebo-controlled multicenter trial. Crit Care Med 1994; 22: 12–21
68. Fisher C J, Dhainaut J F, Opal S M et al. Recombinant human interleukin 1 receptor antagonist in the treatment of patients with sepsis syndrome. JAMA 1994; 271: 1836–1843
69. Knaus W A, Wagner D P, Harrell F E J, Draper E A. What determines prognosis in sepsis? evidence for a comprehensive individual patient risk assessment approach to the design and analysis of clinical trials. In: Reinhart K, Eyrich K, Sprung C (eds) Sepsis. Current Perspectives in Pathophysiology and Therapy. Springer, Berlin, 1994; pp 23–37

70. Preiser J C, Schmartz D, Van der Linden P et al. IL-6 administration has no acute haemodynamic effect in the dog. Cytokine 1991; 3: 1–4
71. Gerard C, Bruyns C, Marchant A, et al. Interleukin 10 reduces the release of tumor necrosis factor and prevents lethality in experimental endotoxemia. J Exp Med 1993; 177: 547–550
72. Marchant A, Vincent J L, Goldman M. The protective role of interleukin-10 in sepsis. In: Vincent J L (ed) Yearbook of Intensive Care and Emergency Medicine – 1994. Springer, Berlin, 1994; pp 42–47
73. Mileski W J, Winn R K, Vedder N B et al. Inhibition of CD-18 dependent neutrophil adherence reduces organ injury after hemorrhagic shock in primates. Surgery 1990; 108: 206–212
74. Vedder N B, Winn R K, Rice C L et al. A monoclonal antibody to the adherence-promoting leukocyte glycoprotein, CD18, reduces organ injury and improves survival from haemorrhagic shock and resuscitation in rabbits. J Clin Invest 1988; 81: 939–944
75. Simpson P J, Todd R F, Fantone J C et al. Reduction of experimental canine myocardial reperfusion injury by a monoclonal antibody (anti-MO1, anti-CD11b) that inhibits leukocyte adhesion. J Clin Invest 1988; 81: 624–629
76. Eichacker P Q, Farese A, Hoffman W D et al. Leukocyte CD11b/18 antigen-directed monoclonal antibody improves early survival and decreases hypoxemia in dogs challenged with tumor necrosis factor. Am Rev Respir Dis 1992; 145: 1023–1029
77. Walsh C J, Carey P D, Cook D J et al. Anti-CD18 antibody attenuates neutropenia and alveolar capillary-membrane injury during gram-negative sepsis. Surgery 1991; 110: 205–212
78. Sharrar S R, Winn R K, Nurry C E et al. A CD 18 monoclonal antibody increases the incidence and severity of subcutaneous abscess formation after high-dose staphylococcus aureus injection in rabbits. Surgery 1991; 110: 213–220
79. Eichacker P Q, Hoffman W D, Farese A et al. Leukocyte CD18 monoclonal antibody worsens endotoxemia and cardiovascular injury in canines with septic shock. J Appl Physiol 1993; 745: 1851–1892
80. Todd R F, Freyer D R. The CD11/18 leukocyte glycoprotein deficiency. Hematol Oncol Clin N Am 1988; 2: 13–31
81. Anderson D C, Schmalsteig F C, Arnaout M A. Abnormalities of polymorphonuclear leukocyte function associated with a heritable deficiency of high molecular weight surface glucoproteins (GP138): Common relationship to diminished cell adherence. J Clin Invest 1989; 74: 536–551
82. Wright S D, Levin S M, Jung M T et al. CR-3 (CD11b/CD18) expresses one binding site for Arg-Gly-Asp containing peptides and a second site for bacterial lipopolysaccharide. J Exp Med 1989; 169: 175–183
83. Snapper J R, Hutchinson A A, Ogletree M L, Brigham K L. Effects of cyclooxygenase inhibitors on the alterations in lung mechanics caused by endotoxemia in the unanesthetized sheep. J Clin Invest 1983; 72: 63–76
84. Winn R, Enderson B, Price S, Rice C L. Indomethacin, but not dazoxiben, reduced lung fluid filtration after E. coli infusion. J Appl Physiol 1988; 64: 2468–2473
85. Zhang H, Benlabed M, Spapen H, Nguyen D N. Prostaglandin E1 increases oxygen extraction capabilities in experimental sepsis. J Surg Res 1994; (in press)
86. Bone R C, Slotman G, Maunder R et al. Randomized double-blind, multicentre study of prostaglandin E1 in patients with the adult respiratory distress syndrome. Chest 1989; 96: 114–119
87. Leeman M, Boeynaems J M, Degaute J P et al. Administration of dazoxiben, a selective thromboxane synthetase inhibibor in patients with adult respiratory distress syndrome. Chest 1984; 87: 726–730
88. Stephenson A H, Lonigro A J, Hyers T M et al. Increased concentrations of leukotrienes in bronchoalveolar lavage fluid of patients with ARDS or at risk for ARDS. Am Rev Respir Dis 1988; 138: 714–719
89. Coggeshall J W, Christman B W, Lefferts P L et al. Effect of inhibition of 5–lipoxygenase metabolism of arachidonic acid on response to endotoxemia in sheep. J Appl Physiol 1988; 65: 1351–1359

90. Benveniste J, Chignard M. A role for PAF-acether (platelet-activating factor) in platelet-dependent vascular diseases? Circulation 1985; 72: 713–717

91. Lefer A M. Induction of tissue injury and altered cardiovascular performance by platelet-activating factor: relevance to multiple systems organ failure. Crit Care Clin 1989; 5: 331–352

92. Inarrea P, Gomez Cambronero J, Pascual J et al. Synthesis of PAF-acether and blood volume changes in Gram-negative sepsis. Immunopharmacology 1985; 9: 45–52

93. Oda M, Satouchi K, Ikeda I et al. The presence of platelet-activating factor associated with eosinophil and/or neutrophil accumulations in the pleural fluids. Am Rev Respir Dis 1990; 141: 1469–1473

94. Chang S W, Feddersen C O, Henson P M, Voelkel N F. Platelet-activating factor mediates haemodynamic changes and lung injury in endotoxin-treated rats. J Clin Invest 1987; 79: 1498–1509

95. Doebber T W, Wu M S, Robbins J C et al. Platelet-activating factor (PAF) involvement in endotoxin-induced hypotension in rats. Studies with PAF-receptor antagonist kadsurenone. Biochem Biophys Res Commun 1985; 127: 799–808

96. Myers A K, Robey J W, Price R M. Relationships between tumour necrosis factor, eicosanoids and platelet-activating factor as mediators of endotoxin-induced shock in mice. Br J Pharmacol 1990; 99: 499–502

97. Sun X M, Hsueh W, Torre Amione G. Effects of in vivo 'priming' on endotoxin-induced hypotension and tissue injury. The role of PAF and tumor necrosis factor. Am J Pathol 1990; 136: 949–956

98. Dhainaut J F, Tenaillon A, Letulzo Y et al. Sepsis Study Group. Efficacy of PAF antagonist (BN52021) in reducing mortality of patients with severe gram-negative sepsis. Circ Shock 1993; 1: 42 (Abstract)

99. Tate R M, Vanbenthuysen K M, Shasby D M, McMurtry I F, Repine J E. Oxygen-radical-mediated permeability oedema and vasoconstriction in isolated perfused rabbit lungs. Am Rev Respir Dis 1982; 126: 802–806

100. Varani J, Fligiel S E, Till G O et al. Pulmonary endothelial cell killing by human neutrophils. Possible involvement of hydroxyl radical. Lab Invest 1985; 53: 656–663

101. Zaslow M C, Clark R A, Stone P J et al. Human neutrophil elastase does not bind to alpha 1–protease inhibitor that has been exposed to activated human neutrophils. Am Rev Respir Dis 1983; 128: 434–439

102. Neuhof H. Actions and interactions of mediators systems and mediators in the pathogenesis of ARDS and multiorgan failure. Acta Anaesthesiol Scand 1991; 35: 7–14

103. Tanswell A K, Freeman B A. Liposome-entrapped antioxidant enzymes prevent lethal O_2 toxicity in the newborn rat. J Appl Physiol 1987; 63: 347–352

104. McMillan D D, Boyd G N. The role of antioxidants and diet in the prevention or treatment of oxygen-induced lung microvascular injury. Ann N Y Acad Sci 1982; 384: 535–543 ·

105. Jackson J H, White C W, McMurtry I F et al. Dimethylthiourea decreases acute lung oedema in phorbol myristate acetate-treated rabbits. J Appl Physiol 1986; 61: 353–360

106. Martin W J, Kachel D L. Reduction of neutrophil-mediated injury to pulmonary endothelial cells by dapsone. Am Rev Respir Dis 1985; 131: 544–547

107. Ward P A, Till G O, Kunkel R, Beauchamp C. Evidence for role of hydroxyl radical in complement and neutrophil-dependent tissue injury. J Clin Invest 1983; 72: 789–801

108. Zhang H, Spapen H, Nguyen D N et al. Protective effects of N-acetylcysteine in endotoxemia. Am J Physiol 1994; 266: H1746–H1754

109. Spies C D, Reinhart K, Witt I et al. Influence of N-acetylcysteine on O_2 consumption and gastric intramucosal pH in septic patients (Abstract). Crit Care Med 1993; 21: S183

110. Granger D L, Hibbs J B, Broadnax L M. Urinary nitrate excretion in relation to murine macrophage activation: Influence of dietary L-arginine and oral NG-monomethyl-L-arginine. J Immunol 1991; 146: 1294–1302

111. Vane J R, Anggard E E, Botting R M. Regulatory functions of the vascular endothelium. N Engl J Med 1990; 323: 27–36

112. Finkel M S, Oddis C V, Jacob T D et al. Negative inotropic effects of cytokines on the heart mediated by nitric oxide. Science 1992; 257: 378–389
113. Estrada C, Gomez C, Martin C et al. Nitric oxide mediates tumor necrosis factor-alpha cytotoxicity in endothelial cells. Biochem Biophys Res Commun 1992; 186: 475–482
114. Nguyen T, Brunson D, Crespi C L et al. DNA damage and mutation in human cells exposed to nitric oxide in vitro. Proc Natl Acad Sci USA 1992; 89: 3030–3034
115. Cobb J P, Natanson C, Hoffman W D et al. N-amino-L-arginine, an inhibitor of nitric oxide synthase, raises vascular resistance but increases mortality rates in awake canines challenged with endotoxin. J Exp Med 1992; 176: 1175–1182
116. Julou-Schaeffer G, Gray G A, Fleming I et al. Loss of vascular responsiveness induced by endotoxin involves L-arginine pathway. Am J Physiol 1990; 259: H1038–H1043
117. Kilbourn R G, Jubran A, Gross S S et al. Reversal of endotoxin-mediated shock by NG-methyl-L-arginine, an inhibitor of nitric oxide synthesis. Biochem Biophys Res Commun 1990; 172: 1132–1138
118. Nava E, Palmer R M, Moncada S. Inhibition of nitric oxide synthesis in septic shock: how much is beneficial? Lancet 1991; 338: 1555–1557
119. Nava E, Palmer R M, Moncada S. The role of nitric oxide in endotoxic shock: Effects of NG-monomethyl-L-arginine. J Cardiovasc Pharmacol 1992; 20: S132–S134
120. Cobb J P, Natanson C, Quezado Z M N et al. Lack of protection by N-Methyl-l-Arginine (NMA), a nitric oxide synthase inhibitor, in endotoxin(LPS)-challenged canines. Crit Care Med 1993; 21: S280
121. Preiser J C, Zhang H, Wachel D et al. Is the endotoxin-induced hypotension related to nitric oxide formation? Eur Surg Res 1994; 26: 10–18
122. Petros A, Bennett D, Vallance P. Effect of nitric oxide synthase inhibitors on hypotension in patients with septic shock. Lancet 1991; 338: 1557–1558
123. Preiser J C, Lejeune P, Roman A et al. Methylene blue administration in septic shock: A clinical trial. Crit Care Med 1995 (in press)
124. Kern J A, Lamb R J, Reed J C et al. Dexamethasone inhibition of interleukin 1 beta production by human monocytes. Posttranscriptional mechanisms. J Clin Invest 1988; 81: 237–244
125. Rees D D, Cellek S, Palmer R M, Moncada S. Dexamethasone prevents the induction by endotoxin of a nitric oxide synthase and the associated effects on vascular tone: An insight into endotoxin shock. Biochem Biophys Res Commun 1990; 173: 541–547
126. Hales C A, Brandstetter R D, Neely C F et al. Methylprednisolone on circulating eicosanoids and vasomotor tone after endotoxin. J Appl Physiol 1986; 61: 185–191
127. The veterans administration systemic sepsis cooperative study group. Effect of high-dose glucocorticoid therapy on mortality in patients with clinical signs of systemic sepsis. N Engl J Med 1987; 317: 659–665
128. Bernard G R, Luce J M, Sprung C L et al. High-dose corticosteroids in patients with the adult respiratory distress syndrome. N Engl J Med 1987; 317: 1565–1570
129. Bone R C, Fisher C J J, Clemmer T P et al. A controlled clinical trial of high-dose methylprednisolone in the treatment of severe sepsis and septic shock. N Engl J Med 1987; 317: 653–658
130. Weigelt J A, Norcross J F, Borman K R, Snyder W H. Early steroid therapy for respiratory failure. Arch Surg 1985; 120: 536–540
131. Golde D W, Baldwin G C. Myeloid growth factors. In: Gallin J L, Goldstein I M, Synderman R (eds) Inflammation: basic principles and clinical correlates. Raven Press, New York, 1992; pp 291–301
132. Nelson S, Summer W, Bagby G et al. Granulocyte colony-stimulating factor enhances pulmonary host defenses in normal and ethanol-treated rats. J Infect Dis 1991; 164: 901–906
133. Eichacker P Q, Waisman Y, Natanson C et al. Recombinant granulocyte colony stimulating factor reduces endotoxemia and improves cardiovascular function and survival during bacterial sepsis in non-neutropenic canines. Clin Res 1993; 41: 24

11

New examinations for anaesthetists

P. B. Hewitt

'Teaching without testing is like cooking without tasting'

(Heard at the Fifth Ottawa Conference, Dundee September 1992)

Completion of postgraduate training in anaesthesia in some parts of the world may be achieved by spending a specified period of time in a training programme which does not include any formal method of assessment. However, no matter how good the standard of practice and education may be in such areas, it must be difficult to prove to the general public that satisfactory standards have been achieved. Lack of formal assessment also removes a significant educational inducement because it is very noticeable that anticipation of formal assessment is a potent stimulus to acquisition of the knowledge and skills which are to be tested.[1] In the United Kingdom there is a strong tradition of postgraduate examinations organized by the Royal Colleges and their Faculties, for the various specialities. This includes the Royal College of Anaesthetists. The European Academy of Anaesthesiology has now been conducting a two-part diploma examination in anaesthesiology and intensive care for more than 10 years and it is gaining increasing importance as an exit examination for training in Europe.

Examinations are used to assess three main attributes of candidates: knowledge, skills and attitudes. Different examination formats are used to assess these three factors. For example, multiple choice question papers can provide reliable tests of factual knowledge but do not provide valid assessment of clinical skills; neither do other forms of written question.[2]

The most valid test of clinical and technical skills may be provided by the candidate's performance in the normal working environment but it is difficult to obtain reliable, unbiased evaluation in these circumstances. Objective structured clinical examinations (OSCEs) have therefore been developed to provide a more reliable method of testing performance of a valid range of clinical and technical skills.[3-5]

Good attitudes and judgmental abilities are very important for safe and effective clinical practice but are difficult to assess. Written questions allow candidates to demonstrate their ability to assign appropriate priorities when discussing management problems and have the advantage of providing lasting evidence of this performance. However, it has been found that marking of essay questions tends to be subjective and varies from examiner to examiner. Oral examinations provide the most effective method of assessing attitudes. However, they need to be guided or structured to reduce the element of chance with variability in topics covered and questioning by different examiners. Training and selective re-appointment of examiners has also been found to improve their performance.[6,7]

In the United Kingdom (UK), University based medical education is linked to hospital based clinical courses, with successful completion of examinations in pathology, medicine, surgery, obstetrics and gynaecology required to achieve medical qualification. This can be a University degree, or, after completion of approved University and hospital clinical courses, achieving success at similar examinations conducted by the Conjoint Boards of the Royal Colleges of Physicians and Surgeons. The medical practitioner must then complete one year of recognized hospital medical and surgical 'preregistration' posts or become a 'fully registered' medical practitioner before starting postgraduate training for a hospital speciality or family (general) practice. In the UK no examination is required for entry into specialist training, but in France an entry examination is required to obtain a place on a hospital training programme.

The functions of examinations depend on their timing in relation to the training period. Most of the UK Royal Colleges hold two-part examinations. The philosophy of the Part 1 examination for Membership of the Royal College of Physicians (MRCP) has been said, in the past, to be elitist,[8] the aim being to identify the best medical graduates in Britain who will go on to a hospital career; high fliers with the intellectual capacity and motivation to become successful consultants in the British Health Service. Traditionally, the first part has been devoted to basic sciences and forms quite a formidable academic hurdle at an early stage of training. The subject matter of this type of 'primary' examination is not directly related to the clinical work undertaken by the trainees at that particular stage of training. It can mean that candidates need to spend some time away from clinical practice in order to undertake formal courses, or work as lecturers in preclinical departments or academic specialities. This performs a certain selection function by requiring possession of the intellectual powers to acquire, and prove, sufficient knowledge of basic sciences relevant to the speciality. However, it does not demonstrate whether the trainee has the required clinical ability or personal attributes.

At a later stage, a second examination is taken to prove the acquisition of appropriate knowledge in the speciality concerned. This may be at the completion of basic specialist training and a requirement for entering higher specialist training, or may be an 'exit' examination at the completion of postgraduate training and a signal of eligibility for independent specialist practice. It is helpful for examiners at a final examination to have a clear concept of what constitutes a minimally competent candidate rather than seeking to differentiate subtle gradations of obscure knowledge or expertise.

The Royal College of Anaesthetists currently conducts a three-part examination. The first part is normally taken after about one year of experience in the speciality and is designed with that level of expertise in mind. It covers the principles of anaesthetic practice (including knowledge of commonly used equipment and the outline of physiology and pharmacology relevant to anaesthesia) plus sufficient knowledge of medicine and surgery to enable a reasonable standard of pre-operative assessment and preparation, and postoperative care. The basic sciences are then examined in detail in the Part 2 examination. This creates a problem if the doctor undertaking postgraduate training finds basic science assessment a hurdle too difficult to surmount when he has already spent a significant period of time in anaesthesia and will be reluctant to embark upon a career change. It also means that the process of education, training and gaining specialist experience is interrupted by this extra hurdle. The Part 3 (Final) examination for the Fellowship of the Royal College of Anaesthetists is taken at the completion of basic specialist training when the doctor will have been medically qualified for at least three years and has spent a minimum of 2 years in recognized anaesthetic training posts. It is *not* an exit examination. Successful candidates are expected to spend a further three years in Higher Specialist Training before being eligible for a Consultant post.

Plans have been prepared to revert to a two-part format in the 1996–97 session. A new-style first-part examination covering basic sciences and clinical skills will be known as the Primary FRCA. This will be attempted between 12 and 18 months of recognized training. The syllabus will include (a) physiology and biochemistry, (b) pharmacology and statistics, (c) physics, clinical measurement and safety, and (d) clinical topics including critical incident analysis. The format will be an objective structured clinical examination (OSCE) and two separate 30-minute *viva voces* (each comprising two 15-minute periods).

The new second-part (Final) examination, leading to the Fellowship of the Royal College of Anaesthetists (FRCA), will include anaesthesia, medicine, intensive therapy, applied aspects of anatomy, physiology, pharmacology and clinical measurement.[9] The Final examination will consist of a multiple choice question (MCQ) paper and a short answer paper. Candidates who are successful in those elements proceed to a 'clinical scenario' viva on the application of basic science to (a) anaesthesia and (b) intensive therapy. This new examination format is expected to have close links with the new training arrangements as described in the Royal College of Anaesthetists' document 'Specialist Training in Anaesthesia, Supervision and Assessment'.[10] It is anticipated that successful completion of the Primary will be required before a trainee can enter the new unified training grade (to be called a 'specialist registrar') and completion of the FRCA (second part examination) as a requirement for proceeding to the fifth year of training.

The current Part 3 (Final) examination covers all aspects of anaesthetic practice and is tested by a multiple choice question paper, a written question (essay) paper, a clinical examination and two oral examinations, one of which is structured and the other free-ranging. During 1994 the clinical examination was changed from the traditional 'long case' format to an objective structured clinical examination (OSCE) format. In the traditional 'long case' format, the candidate had 30 minutes to take a history and perform physical examination on a volunteer patient. This was followed by a 25 minute discussion of the case with an examiner plus analysis of other material such as radiographs and electrocardiographs. The OSCE tests a wider range of clinical and technical skills.

THE OBJECTIVE STRUCTURED CLINICAL EXAMINATION (OSCE)

Structured clinical examinations were developed in the 1970s to overcome the problems associated with traditional clinical examinations.[3-5,11] The OSCE is an examination structure in which candidates are assessed at a series of short 'stations', or booths, with one or more aspects of competence being tested at each station. This format allows a wider range of skills to be assessed during the course of the examination. The candidate's performance is observed by the examiners rather than being conducted out of sight of the assessors as often happened with the traditional 'long case' clinical examination. The examiners remain at their stations while the candidates move round the circuit. Consequently, each candidate is assessed carrying out the same clinical exercises by the same examiners using checklists for marking. Some medical schools have been using OSCEs for 15 years.[3-5,11-13] The traditional clinical examination has been largely discredited on the grounds of poor reliability and the structured clinical examination seems to be a very credible alternative.[3,6,12-15]

The OSCE in the Part 3 FRCA examination consists of twelve stations. The candidates rotate, spending five minutes at each station with a 1.5 minute changeover time between each. Some stations are linked 'follow-on' stations where questions relevant to information gained at the previous one can be pursued in greater detail. Two circuits are run in parallel to increase the number of candidates examined per day.

The aspects covered by the Part 3 OSCE are outlined in a Skills Directory prepared by the Royal College of Anaesthetists.[16] Many of the traditional skills such as taking a medical history, physical examination, data interpretation and problem solving continue to be tested but in a more structured way than previously. The exercises involved are more focussed in order to fit into the five minute time slots and ensure that the same tasks are undertaken by successive candidates. For the first time in a United Kingdom postgraduate examination 'standardized patients' who present reproducible clinical histories are being used. Some aspect of resuscitation skills is evaluated with each candidate and basic life support technique observed.

The Skills Directory is divided under four main headings: (a) Clinical Assessment (including history and physical examination), (b) Data Interpretation (including clinical, radiological and laboratory data), (c) Communication Skills (including obtaining consent, explanation of pre- and postoperative care and intensive care to patients and relatives and giving instructions to nurses), and (d) Technical skills (including clinical procedures and safe use of equipment). The Skills Directory will continue to develop in line with changes in training and practice.

Marking is carried out according to predetermined guidelines using agreed checklists. Subjective bias is minimized by assessing each group of candidates during the day on the same set of stations and using comparable stations covering the same types of skills on succeeding days. This format will allow feedback to candidates in greater detail than previously in order to reveal areas where skills did not reach the required standard.

STANDARDIZED PATIENTS

Standardized patients, who may also be referred to as 'simulated patients' or 'SPs', were first introduced in North America in the early 1960s when they were called 'programmed patients'.[17] An 'SP' can be defined as a person who has been coached to simulate an actual patient so accurately that the simulation cannot be detected by a skilled clinician. They may be chronic, stable patients with reliable physical signs; specially trained full-time teachers/assessors; professional actors or role-players; or any intelligent layman who has been appropriately briefed. Their use means that it is possible for a whole group of candidates to be presented with the same test scenarios for evaluation of their clinical skills thus facilitating greater consistency in assessment. They are being used to an increasing extent both for teaching medical students and as subjects for clinical examinations for assessment of history taking, physical examination and communication skills. In the USA they are used extensively both for teaching and for the licensing examinations.[8-21] In the United Kingdom organisations such as the Casualties Union provide volunteers who create impressive simulations for training and testing, e.g. the St. John's Ambulance Brigade in the management of accidents.

MULTIPLE CHOICE QUESTIONS (MCQs)

Although these are technically reliable they cannot be regarded as a valid method for testing clinical ability.[22] The simplest format in current use uses a single stem and multiple 'True-False' options. Marks are obtained for correct answers, deducted for incorrect answers (negative marking) and no marks given for registering 'don't know'. 'Marker' questions can be employed to indicate the performance level of a group of candidates relative to previous groups in order to establish the overall pass mark at a consistent level. Other forms of multiple choice questions can be set e.g. making best matches from multiple options which are designed to reduce the 'cueing effect' of the question format and to minimize the opportunity of gaining marks through intelligent, or intuitive, guesswork.

THE ORAL EXAMINATION

There is widespread use of oral (or *viva voce*) examinations in the speciality of anaesthesia throughout the English speaking world.[23,24] They aim to evaluate not only the candidate's knowledge but also, more importantly, the ability to 'problem solve' and to communicate, or conduct an intelligent dialogue, on a professional topic. Reliability can be affected by factors relating to the examiner, the candidate and the exact format of the examination. Therefore, care is required to prepare appropriately constructed questions. During oral examinations (as well as exploring the extent of the candidate's knowledge, e.g. of basic sciences related to anaesthesia, etc.), evaluation of clinical situations, choices of techniques and agents, ability to deal with emergency situations, decision making and communication skills are all involved. This wide potential contributes to the validity of oral examinations but leads to difficulty in making reliable evaluation of a candidate. There is no direct permanent record of the candidate's performance therefore subsequent reassessment is difficult.

Care has to be taken to reduce the subjective element in marking. This is helped by structuring questions so that all candidates are led down similar pathways and cover similar subject matter. Furthermore, when clinical scenarios are used they should be clear and simple without an excess of complicating factors which cannot be dealt with in the time available. It is helpful for the examination team to have devised a decision tree beforehand so that guidance can be given to examiners on the major points which should be covered to attain satisfactory marks. In some scenarios, emergency situations may be introduced to ascertain whether the candidate can react quickly and make a series of appropriate decisions. Such questions are perceived to be stressful for candidates.

Oral examinations are conducted using a minimum of two examiners for each candidate. One examiner asks the question while the other notes the aspects covered and any special points that will be important to consider when allocating marks. It is then usual for the roles to be exchanged for the second half of the *viva voce*. Both examiners should then independently evaluate the candidate's performance before conferring to award an agreed mark. Examination committees can keep records of the marks awarded by individual examiners, as well as the final agreed marks, in order to assess the performances of the examiners. These records can then be used to find out whether some examiners tend to award lower marks (the 'hawks') or higher marks (the 'doves') than their colleagues. They can also see whether, on the occasions where the individual marks differ, the agreed marks are at the higher or lower levels and enable any instances where the two examiners award widely separated marks to be investigated. It is helpful to have a third examiner or 'observer' present for all or some of the oral examinations to evaluate the conduct and standard of the examination and the marking then provide relevant feedback to examiners and examination committees. Examiners who do not perform consistently may not be re-appointed.[6]

IN-TRAINING ASSESSMENT

In-training evaluations can be used to assess various components of competence including clinical and technical skills, problem solving and interpersonal skills within a normal working environment. In this respect, they could be regarded as the most valid way of assessing whether an anaesthetist is performing the tasks undertaken in his everyday work to a satisfactory and safe standard. The major problem, however, is the difficulty of ensuring comparable standards at different centres. This format is used for the final in-training evaluation report (FITER) which is completed for each candidate, by their programme director, when they are finishing their speciality training for the Royal Colleges of Physicians and Surgeons of Canada examination.

FORMATIVE ASSESSMENT AND SUMMATIVE ASSESSMENT

Examinations can also be used during the training period to help the trainee assess progress, to find out whether knowledge and performance has improved over a period of training and experience and find out how the educational standard achieved compares with contemporaries or with candidates sitting the actual examinations. This type of formative assessment is being provided by the European Academy of Anaesthesiology which allows anaesthetists in training to sit the same multiple choice question papers as the candidates and provides feedback on how their performance compares with that of the candidates and those at the same stage of training. The feedback is subdivided into the various areas of questioning to give the trainees helpful guidance on their strengths and weaknesses. Thus formative assessment can provide anaesthetists in training with information as to their progress and achievements and provides motivation for study before they undertake their summative assessment.

VALIDITY AND RELIABILITY

The validity of a test is the degree to which it measures what it is supposed to measure.[4,25] For example, a valid clinical examination should cover the ability to obtain a relevant history from a patient, carry out a physical examination, identify the problems, reach a diagnosis, identify appropriate investigations and recommend and carry out clinical, technical and communication skills.[4,16]

Reliability is a measure of the reproducibility of an examination, or the consistency and precision with which it tests what it is supposed to test. For example, a well-designed multiple choice question paper can provide a very reliable (reproducible) test of knowledge.

Unfortunately, the tests which are most easily reproducible may be those which are less relevant to clinical practices while the tests which most closely resemble important skills can be difficult to mark objectively.[26,27] Constant efforts are made to eliminate variability due to differences between different examiners, different patients used as examination subjects or tests carried out on different days. This is where structured clinical examinations using standardized patients can help to make clinical examinations more reliable (reproducible) while testing a wide range of clinical and technical skills to ensure that they are also relevant and valid.

OTHER 'EXAMINATIONS' FOR ANAESTHETISTS

Many anaesthetists are extensively involved in resuscitation and care of patients who have suffered major trauma. In these areas they are coping with acute emergency situations together with a team of professionals with different speciality backgrounds, training and attitudes. In order to function effectively as a team it is vital that all concerned are familiar with a common core of knowledge, skills and protocols. In order to achieve such teamwork many anaesthetists are now undertaking courses in Advanced Trauma Life Support (ATLS), Advanced Life Support (ALS) (renamed Advanced Cardiac Life Support) and Advanced Paediatric Life Support (APLS). These intensive course are followed by tests using simulated accident victims and candidates achieving high marks can subsequently attend futher courses to become trainers themselves. This system, started in the USA, is achieving standards which are beginning to be accepted internationally.

CONCLUSIONS

No one method of examination is ideal and the perfect test will never be attained. Testing is required to ascertain the abilities of entrants to the speciality to become competent and safe anaesthetists, to provide formative assessment during training and to give an indication that adequate knowledge and skills have been acquired and appropriate attitudes developed for a specialist to be accredited as suitable to practice without requiring supervision. The syllabuses prepared for the examinations and the methods used for assessing them should also provide a constructive stimulus for effective learning. After completing the required examinations, peer review and continuing medical education will be required to ensure that the standard of performance in clinical practice is maintained and continues to develop along with advances in anaesthesia.

REFERENCES

1. Newble D I, Jaeger K. The effect of assessments and examinations on the learning of medical students. Medical Education 1983; 17: 165–171
2. Lowry S. Medical Education: Assessment of students. BMJ 1993; 306; 51–54
3. Harden R M, Stevenson M, Downie W W, Wilson G M. Assessment of clinical competence using objective structured examination. BMJ 1975; 1: 447–451
4. Harden R M, Gleeson F A. Assessment of medical competence using an objective structured clinical examination (OSCE). ASME Medical Education Booklet No. 8 Medical Education 1979; 13: 39–54
5. Cuschieri A, Gleeson F A, Harden R M, Wood R A B. A new approach to a final examination in surgery. Annals of the Royal College of Surgeons of England 1979; 61: 400–405
6. Newble D I, Hoare J, Sheldrake P F. The selection and training of examiners for clinical examinations. Medical Education 1980; 14: 345–349
7. Vickers M D. Quality assurance in postgraduate examinations. In: Zorab J S M, Vickers M D, Harmer M (eds), Baillière's Clinical Anaesthesiology 8 (iii): Basic Principles of Education and Training. Baillière Tindall, London, 1994: pp 711–726
8. Medical Practice: Symposium. MRCP: 1977. B M J 1978; 1: 217–220
9. The Royal College of Anaesthetists's Examination Committee. The two-part fellowship examination in anaesthetics. Royal College of Anaesthetists, Newsletter 1994 (October); 19: 6
10. The Royal College of Anaesthetists. Specialist training in anaesthesia, supervision and assessment. London: Royal College of Anaesthetists. 1994
11. Newble D I, Elmslie R G. A new approach to the final examinations in medicine and surgery. Lancet 1981; 2: 517–518
12. Newble D I. Eight years' experience with a structured clinical examination. Medical Education 1988; 22: 200–204
13. Hart I R, Harden R M, DesMarchais J. Current Development in Assessing Clinical Competence. Canadian Health, Montreal, 1992
14. Newble D I, Hoare, J, Elmislie R G. The validity and reliability of a new examination of clinical competence of medical students. Medical Education 1981; 15: 46–52
15. Newble D I. Improving the clinical and oral examination process. In: Hart I R, Harden R M (eds) Further developments in Clinical Competence. Can Health Publs, Montreal, 1987
16. The Royal College of Anaesthetists. OSCE (Objective Structured Clinical Examination) Part 3 FRCA. 1993
17. Norman G R, Barrows H S, Gliva G, Woodward C. Simulated patients. In: Neufeld V R, Norman G R, (eds). Assessing Clinical Competence. Springer, New York, 1985
18. Stillman P I, Swanson D, Regan M B et al. Assessment of clinical skills of residents utilizing standardized patients. Ann Int Med 1991; 114: 393–401
19. Tamblyn R M, Klass D J, Scnabl G K, Kopelow M L. The accuracy of standardized patient presentations. Medical Education 1991; 25: 100–109
20. Swanson D B, Norcini J J. Factors influencing reproducibility of tests using standardized patients. Teach Learn Med 1989; 1: 158–166
21. Van der Vleuten C P M, Swanson D B. Assessment of clinical skills using standardized patients: state of the art. Teach Learn Med 1990; 2: 58–76
22. Newble D I, Baxter A, Elmslie R G. A comparison of multiple choice tests and free-response tests in examinations of clinical competence. Medical Education 1979; 13: 263–268
23. Pope W D B. Anaesthesia oral examination. Can J Anaesth 1993; 40: 907–910
24. Eagle C J. Martineau R, Hamilton K. The oral examination in anaesthetic resident evaluation. Can J Anaesth 1993; 40: 947–953
25. Neufeld V R. introduction to measurement properties. In: Neufeld R V, Norman G R (eds). Assessing Clinical Competence. Springer, New York, 1985; 45

26. Van der Vleuten C P M, Norman G R, De Graaff E. Pitfalls in the pursuit of objectivity: issues of reliability. Medical Education 1991; 25: 110–118
27. Norman G R, Van der Vleuten C P M, De Graaff E. Pitfalls in the pursuit of objectivity: issuses of validity, efficiency and acceptability. Medical Education 1991; 25: 119–126

Index